Series on Technology
and Social Priorities

NATIONAL ACADEMY
OF ENGINEERING

INSTITUTE OF MEDICINE

New
Medical
Devices

Invention, Development,
and Use

Karen B. Ekelman
Editor

NATIONAL ACADEMY PRESS
Washington, D.C. 1988

National Academy Press   **2101 Constitution Avenue, NW**   **Washington, DC 20418**

The National Academy of Engineering was established in 1964, under the charter of the National Academy of Sciences, as a parallel organization of outstanding engineers. It is autonomous in its administration and in the selection of its members, sharing with the National Academy of Sciences the responsibility for advising the federal government. The National Academy of Engineering also sponsors engineering programs aimed at meeting national needs, encourages education and research, and recognizes the superior achievements of engineers. Dr. Robert M. White is president of the National Academy of Engineering.

The Institute of Medicine was chartered in 1970 by the National Academy of Sciences to enlist distinguished members of the appropriate professions in the examination of policy matters pertaining to the health of the public. In this, the Institute acts under both the Academy's 1983 congressional charter responsibility to be an adviser to the federal government and its own initiative in identifying issues of medical care, research, and education. Samuel O. Thier is president of the Institute of Medicine.

This publication has been reviewed by a group other than the authors according to procedures approved by a Report Review Committee. The interpretations and conclusions in this publication are those of the authors and do not purport to represent the views of the councils, officers, or staff of the National Academy of Engineering or the Institute of Medicine.

Funds for the National Academy of Engineering's Symposium Series on Technology and Social Priorities are provided by the Andrew W. Mellon Foundation, Carnegie Corporation of New York, and the Academy's Technology Agenda Program.

Library of Congress Cataloging-in-Publication Data

New medical devices: factors influencing invention, development, and
  use/Karen B. Ekelman, editor.
     p.   cm.—(Series on technology and social priorities)
   At head of title: National Academy of Engineering; Institute of
Medicine.
   Based on a symposium held at the National Academy of Sciences,
Washington, D.C., Mar. 9–10, 1987.
   Includes index.
   ISBN 0-309-03847-2.   ISBN 0-309-03846-4 (pbk.)
   1. Medical instruments and apparatus—Evaluation—Congresses.
2. Medical innovations—Economic aspects—Congresses.   I. Ekelman,
Karen B.   II. National Academy of Engineering.   III. Institute of
Medicine (U.S.)   IV. Series.
   [DNLM: 1. Equipment and supplies—congresses.   W 26 N532 1987]
R856.A2N495 1988
610' .28—dc19
DNLM/DLC   88-12580
for Library of Congress   CIP

Printed in the United States of America

SYMPOSIUM ADVISORY COMITTEE

Cochairmen

ROBERT W. MANN, Massachusetts Institute of Technology
WALTER L. ROBB, General Electric Company

Members

J. D. ANDRADE, University of Utah
SUSAN BARTLETT FOOTE, University of California, Berkeley
JOHN H. GIBBONS, Office of Technology Assessment, U.S. Congress
RUTH S. HANFT, George Washington University
PETER BARTON HUTT, Covington and Burling, Washington, D.C.
WILLIAM W. LOWRANCE, The Rockefeller University
LARRY MIIKE, Office of Technology Assessment, U.S. Congress
FREDERICK C. ROBBINS, Case Western University
GEORGE E. THIBAULT, Massachusetts General Hospital

Staff

KAREN B. EKELMAN, *NAE Fellow*
NANCY B. ISENBERG, *NAE Fellow*

Foreword

The impressive breadth and comprehensiveness of the collective contributions to the symposium on which this book is based preclude any but a sharp focus for these foreword comments. But if a single word had to stand for the conference, and for what this professor wished to emphasize, it would be "interdisciplinary."

The dynamic of the meeting, inevitably restrained in printed form, is indebted to the informed presentations and vigorous discussions of the participants and to the committee and staff who designed the program. We ranged over the device spectrum from origin to obsolescence and heard from representatives of numerous university departments and professional schools and spokespersons from industry, finance, government, and the several customers—physicians and hospitals. Again invoking personal experience, I concentrate on the innovation stage of an intrinsically interdisciplinary process.

Samuel Thier, in his thoughtful and candid overview, elects to focus on the scientific base of medical devices. But that historic source of innovation seemed of little relevancy in the engaging stories of the determined and pragmatic inventors. Edward Roberts expressed a similar view in his conclusion that "innovation in medical devices is usually based on engineering problem solving by individuals or small firms, is often incremental rather than radical, seldom depends on the results of long-term research in the basic sciences, and generally does not reflect the recent generation of fundamental new knowledge." Frank Samuel coalesces both positions—that of the inventors and of management science—by asserting, "We cannot worry very effectively about the discovery of new knowledge. . . .'' From the perspective of government, Louise Russell agreed with Anthony Romeo's conclusion that increased federal funding for research is not warranted at present, although Dr. Romeo did note that "R&D is an investment [that] depends heavily on the federal government" and that "private industry cannot be relied on to do basic research." William Lowrance observes in his summarizing remarks, "We should not feel too bad about the accomplishment so far" and "few if any lines of medical technology development have been stifled." He notes that "unlike Chrysler, the steel manufacturers, and the railroads, the medical manufacturers . . . have not begged for federal bailout or special treatment."

On the issues of the national economy and international competitiveness, I would argue that medical technology could easily experience the same wearisome decline endemic now across so many once American-dominated product lines. The assaults will come both from lower-cost replication from the Pacific Rim nations and from international competitors who do invest in R&D and successfully manage technology transfer. The ultrasound lithotriptor, a device that obviates the hazards and long hospital recovery periods associated with surgical removal of gall stones, is produced in the Federal Republic of Germany, where it emerged from research on the effects of hailstones on aircraft. We are seeing cochlear implants of superior effectiveness based on Australian research. Philips A. G. of the Netherlands, which supplements its consumer electronics products with medical technology, tops in dollar volume all comparable Japanese firms exporting to the United States. So, whatever the economic and regulatory tensions we experience in this country, we had best not rest on our R&D oars lest medical devices join the decline of U.S. automobiles, steel, and railroads.

In my opinion, the research areas grievously underserved are interdisciplinary questions undergirding future medical devices. We have run the string of devices nostalgically described by our inventors. Future medical technology will increasingly require more fundamental understanding at the organ, cell, and subcellular levels, and it will be based on collaborative biological and physical science research. Leo Thomas, in his review of the study mandated by the National Science Foundation (NSF), outlines a number of such areas—biomaterials, biosensors, artificial organs, functional neurostimulation. All of these topics deal intimately with the biological state but address questions framed largely in physical science and engineering terms. Such nonparochial research is not likely to be done anywhere but in a university setting, but even here traditional department organization frequently impedes the essential collaboration among persons skilled in their respective realms.

Even more disturbing to this observer is the accelerating trend toward biological research focusing heavily, if not exclusively, at the molecular level. Physics has traditionally taken a reductionist view of science, and biologists are following that pathway—admittedly with great success. Left vacant, however, are vast research areas of interest and promise at the subcellular, cellular, and organ levels where neither biologists nor physicists and engineers alone are well equipped to frame and address important questions. The artificial heart program—however its economic and social viability are assessed—could be a paradigm of this dilemma. The problem of long-term biomaterial blood compatibility, obvious two decades ago, still severely limits longevity. How to control a replacement heart in a physiologically appropriate manner has hardly been addressed. How the wear and tear of articular cartilage, the clinical sign of osteoarthritis, develops—whether by a purely mechanical process, a purely biological process, or a combination of the two—is an open question despite the wide prevalence and expensive morbidity of the disease, and thus far, too narrowly focused research. A myriad of similar questions can be posed at the interface between physics and biology—some to explicate pathology where devices may prove inappropriate; others to lay firm foundations on which to develop new technology.

The awareness of this interdisciplinary knowledge gap and its significance is just beginning to be discerned. Sigma Xi's recent centennial report, *A New Agenda for Science*, stresses the need for, and opportunities in, "interdisciplinary science." Leo Thomas describes in this volume the National Research Council (NRC) Engineering Research Board study sponsored by NSF. The National Academies of Sciences and Engineering and the Institute of Medicine jointly have sponsored a government-university-industry research roundtable entitled "Multidisciplinary Research and Education Programs in Universities: Making Them Work." NSF has just announced a new initiative in "Emerging Technologies" with "Tissue Engineering" among its first two targets, and the Institute of Medicine has joined with the Commission on Physical Sciences, Mathematics, and Resources of the NRC in a Committee on Fostering Research Collaboration Among the Physical and Engineering Sciences and the Biological and Clinical Sciences.

University departmental faculty organization and curricula pedagogy tend to "parochialize nature." These new initiatives in interdisciplinary science must identify and promote new models for the conduct of research essential to the undergirding of future medical technology. On a longer time frame, but even more vital, they must develop the educational strategies necessary to equip humans with the rigor of the several underlying disciplines, coupled with the skills and perspectives to attack problems which promote, regain, and extend human health.

ROBERT W. MANN
Cochairman
Symposium Advisory Committee

In an era when virtually every discussion of U.S. technology relates to concern over our slipping global position, it is good to see the National Academy of Engineering and the Institute of Medicine examine the complexities of a U.S. success story: medical devices, a market in which the nation has both the technical and manufacturing lead. Admittedly our nation has the highest level of use of such devices and the correspondingly highest cost, but they help give us the best and most widely available health care in the world. Although we have not invented all the winning products, we have a reasonable share, and we have responded effectively to interventions made elsewhere.

The United States has done well, and done it in diverse ways: through the efforts of entrepreneurs, through developments carried out by big companies, and through collaboration between university and industry. That diversity of successful approaches makes for complications. But it also gives our system a hybrid vigor that it might otherwise lack. As long as we do not destroy any of these complementary routes, the U.S. system of medical device innovation should remain strong.

We should not, however, complacently assume that the future will remain the same as the past. In the next generation of innovation, the emphasis may be on lowering cost and increasing ease of use, rather than providing wholly new diagnostic modes or major performance improvements in existing ones. Such an emphasis on productivity and effectiveness might favor overseas rivals who have excelled in lower cost, higher quality design in other fields. We could lose our industrial position in spite of a continuing strength in research and invention, improved specifications, or even new capabilities.

So the future presents both positives and negatives. On the plus side, the United States will remain the number one market for medical diagnostic equipment because of our nation's willingness to fund a high level of health care, the strength of our medical professions, and our excellent medical schools. And we retain a range of companies eager to serve that market.

On the minus side must be counted our litigious society; the difficulty of making objective health care assessments that will define when devices are really cost effective; and those past weaknesses in cost- and quality-conscious manufacturing, which U.S. industries are now overcoming, but perhaps not fast enough.

In the light of these uncertainties, and given the complexity of the problems, it is not surprising that the conference on which this book is based had difficulty in coming up with crisp conclusions or recommendations. But William Lowrance has provided a set of "Summarizing Reflections" that ought to be required reading for anyone in, or preparing to enter, the medical equipment business. What a complex field—yet, for one who has been there, what an exciting and satisfying field!

So may this compilation of the conference not scare away aspiring scientist-physician-entrepreneur-businessmen. Rather, may it increase their knowledge, stimulate their ambition, excite their senses, and, above all, help ensure the continuance of strong U.S. leadership in the development, sales, and proper use of medical devices.

WALTER L. ROBB
Cochairman
Symposium Advisory Committee

Preface and Acknowledgments

Scientifically based disease prevention and health promotion have been made possible by the numerous scientific and technological advances that have redefined medicine in the twentieth century. One of the important influences in this process is the subject of this volume, the development and use of new medical devices.

As in other areas of technological advance, the benefits of new medical devices are not without cost and raise many issues for study. We know, as Samuel O. Thier, president of the Institute of Medicine, points out in this book, that certain medical devices, such as the computed tomographic scanner, have reduced the net cost of treating some diseases. But how are other new technologies related to the rising cost of health care, and how can we ensure the most cost-effective use of new equipment? How can we promote innovation in medical technologies when the trends in the judicial application of tort law have made industries hesitant to develop products for which profits may be modest and liabilities severe?

To explore these important issues and better understand the inter-relationship of engineering, medicine, invention, and public policy, the National Academy of Engineering (NAE) and the Institute of Medicine (IOM) jointly convened the symposium "New Medical Devices: Factors Influencing Invention, Development, and Use" on March 3–4, 1987. The symposium brought physicians, engineers, and scientists together with industry executives, lawyers, ethicists, economists, and government officials to explore key factors that will influence development and use of innovative medical devices during the next decade. Symposium participants identified current trends in federal and private support of technological innovation, medical device regulation, product liability, and health care reimbursement. In addition, participants addressed important general issues, such as how to sustain technological innovation and health care quality in a rapidly changing health care environment and how to encourage and support inventors.

After a highly successful symposium characterized by discussion that was as fruitful and wide-ranging as would be expected of a diverse and knowledgeable assembly, we set about transforming the presentations and discussion into their present form. The symposium considered topics in three general areas, which make up the three major divisions of this volume. These topics are (1) innovation and use of new medical devices; (2) current trends in federal and private support of technological innovation, medical device regulation, product liability, and health care reimbursement; and (3) several perspectives on how these trends interact to influence the availability and appropriate use of new medical devices.

The symposium and this volume are particularly noteworthy in that they represent the first major collaborative effort undertaken by the NAE and the IOM. This activity could not have been completed successfully without such collaboration, and I would like especially to thank Samuel O. Thier and Frederick C. Robbins, current and former IOM presidents, respectively, for their continued enthusiasm and support for this project.

We are indebted to John H. Gibbons and Larry Miike of the congressional Office of Technology Assessment for making available to us in draft form a collection of vignettes in which a number of inventors described their experience in the innovation process for specific medical technologies. This book includes five of these vignettes by inventors whose personal presentations at the symposium were among its high points.

Many people contributed to the success of the symposium and to the publication of this volume. I would like especially to thank cochairmen Robert W. Mann and Walter L. Robb and the other members of the symposium advisory committee: J. D. Andrade, Susan Bartlett Foote, John H. Gibbons, Ruth S. Hanft, Peter Barton Hutt, William W. Lowrance, Larry Miike, and George E. Thibault. Special appreciation is due to Karen B. Ekelman, NAE Fellow, who served as staff director for the symposium and editor of this volume. Thanks are also due to the many people in the NAE and the IOM who played constructive roles, including Caroline G. Anderson, Jesse H. Ausubel, Enriqueta C. Bond, Penelope J. Gibbs, Clifford S. Goodman, Karen B. Ekelman, Nancy B. Isenberg, H. Dale Langford, Sandra H. Matthews, and Wallace K. Waterfall.

ROBERT M. WHITE
President
National Academy of Engineering

Contents

xiii

New
Medical
Devices

Part 1
Medical Device Innovation and Health Care

New Medical Devices
and Health Care

SAMUEL O. THIER

The purpose of this book is to describe how somebody comes up with an idea for a medical device, develops it, and tests it; how it is regulated and marketed; how it is introduced; and then how it serves the purposes of health care. Although it is easy to believe that the device is the primary concern, it is my intent to caution against that perspective. Medical devices, no matter how innovative, are means to an end. The end, of course, is prevention of disease, correction of disease, and rehabilitation from disease.

Those who are involved in the development of medical devices and want to have them used properly must be extremely frustrated by the fact that devices often are blamed for the rising cost of health care. Yet, it is impossible to imagine anybody practicing medicine today without medical devices and medical technology. Why is it that we have a dependence on technology for skilled practice and at the same time a resistance to technology? I think there are several types of reasons—cultural, economic, and scientific. I will quickly scan the first two and then focus a bit more on the scientific base of medical devices.

The problem in introducing new technology is an old one. For example, a newspaper editorial in 1834 said of a medical instrument: "That it will ever come into general use, notwithstanding its value, is extremely doubtful because its beneficial application requires much time and gives a good bit of trouble, both to the patient and the practitioner because its hue and character are foreign and opposed to all our habits and associations. There is something even ludicrous in

3

the picture of a gray physician proudly listening through a long tube applied to the patient's thorax'' (McKusick, 1958). That *London Times* editorial was criticizing the introduction of the stethoscope. New medical technologies since then have also been resisted, sometimes by the public, sometimes by the profession, sometimes by both.

In general, the medical profession is a very conservative group and does not accept new technologies readily. That is not all bad. Readers of the *New England Journal of Medicine* and the *Journal of the American Medical Association* (*JAMA*) every week see reports about the introduction of some new technology, some new test, something that will advance the way in which we practice medicine. If we were to change according to each of those reports, we would end up changing directions like Ping-Pong balls, and our use of technology would be ludicrous.

One of the tensions in the system is between the natural resistance to new technology and the fascinated attraction to it. That emotional ambivalence is an important reality. But there is a more important economic resistance: technology generally and devices particularly have become identified as culprits in the rise of health care costs. The general sense is that every time a new technology is introduced, the costs of care are driven up. That may be true if the technology is expensive and is used often.

However, technology also can lower costs in many health care circumstances. Sometimes the cost-cutting effect is direct and obvious. Other times it is indirect, measurable mainly in the quicker return of patients to a productive existence, which rarely is calculated in the costs of introducing medical technology.

Some of the stigma on technology as costly stems from its improper siting. Because of the health care reimbursement system, we have commonly put technology in the most expensive settings, where the support staff and overhead costs are the highest. Other blame attaches to our failure to ensure skilled use of the technology. The assumption that we could release technology on an unprepared medical profession and have it spread with appropriate skills throughout the nation is a delusion. That simply does not happen, and thus we have persons applying technologies who are prepared neither by skill nor by knowledge of the proper indications for use. A further problem relates to a system that pays practitioners more for technologic skills than for cognitive medical skills. When that happens, it drives the use of technology into inappropriate applications.

Something I wrote a few years ago puts it in perspective from the physician's standpoint.

It is a paradox of modern medicine that, as technology provides for greater precision in diagnosis and treatment, practicing physicians are becoming less critical and efficient in its use. The difficulties for the physician in practice are understandable. The last two to three decades have been historically unique in the rate at which new biomedical knowledge has been produced and applied. New insights into the basic mechanism of disease have been translated into new diagnostic tests and therapeutic modalities. . . . New technology is frequently introduced through journal articles, consultants' suggestions, conferences, postgraduate courses, and newsletters. Often there is inadequate perspective provided for the use of the technology and certainly inadequate perspective in a clinical circumstance or in relation to other existing technologies.

The physician, understandably, continues to use what has proven helpful in the past and merely adds new technology to established patterns. The result is a proliferation of technology rather than substitution of newer and better approaches for outdated ones (Thier, 1983).

What are we to do in response to burgeoning innovation? It does not permit time for assimilation of the information that would enable us to make proper use of the technology and ensure that patients will benefit to the maximum extent possible from innovation. The way in which we deal with technology does not permit focused analysis of how good it is and how well it works, nor does it permit effective long-range monitoring of who uses it and how well they use it.

In the assessment of medical technology there are several perspectives that must be satisfied. The needs of somebody who is pondering reimbursement for a technology differ considerably from the needs of a hospital deciding whether it wishes to introduce the technology for the care of its patients. That information, in turn, differs from what physicians need to know to change their practice patterns and use the technology, and that differs from what a patient needs to know to ask proper questions of the doctor.

I would like to suggest a framework for introducing technology that will enable us to determine where that technology fits in the scheme of things and what its contribution to health care might be. The perspective is that of the health profession, the people conducting screening for, and prevention of, disease and employing diagnostic technology, therapeutic technology, and rehabilitative technology.

The development of health care in the past century first emphasized diagnosis, because it was something a physician could actually do. Much later came the methods of effective therapy that currently get so much attention. The discovery of, and investment in, good screening techniques and in major rehabilitative measures is recent, but it is probably much more important economically than the diagnostic and therapeutic modalities. The result of this developmental history is that the reimbursement system has been focused on diagnosis and therapy instead of screening and rehabilitation.

SCREENING

Screening has both positive and negative aspects. A good example of a positive screening technology is the test for AIDS virus antibody. The test had two major goals initially. One was to protect the blood supply and the other was to provide epidemiologic information. Its theoretical strength in protecting the blood supply was quickly proven. Because the procedure was readily developed, inexpensive, broadly applicable, accurate, and became more accurate in practice, it represented a superb screening test. However, when screening tests go beyond something as focused as protecting the blood supply to screening populations for AIDS—a fatal, incurable disease with social stigmas—questions of individual rights versus protection of the public are raised. False-positive results that have little effect on protection of the blood supply become a major concern in screening populations with a low incidence of the disease. The AIDS virus antibody test protected a resource, provided excellent epidemiologic information, was inexpensive, and will have an enormous payback, because it will be done over and over again for years to come in ever-larger segments of the population. That makes it a very successful technology.

For an example of a potentially negative side of screening, there is mammography—a superb test. It enables us to identify a lesion in a woman's breast at a very early stage. A pioneering controlled clinical trial demonstrated that, in women over age 50, mammography could reveal lesions sufficiently early for successful therapeutic intervention. In those women, mammographic screening was cost-effective.

As the technology improved, the dose of radiation was lowered, the pictures were of better quality, and several logical assumptions were made. One was that if the procedure could be performed at a lower dose and if it was more accurate, it could be applied to a larger population of women, which would increase the benefits. Therefore, the screening was applied in a demonstration project to women less than 50 years old. But the test is not without risk, particularly in younger women. Also, we are still debating the effects of radiation at low dose.

Thus, we now had a risk without a documented benefit. The entire issue became exceedingly heated. The debate cast doubt on the very effective screening for women over age 50, confused women completely as to whether mammography was good or bad, drove them away from diagnostic mammography for which there was no question of benefit, and created havoc. The reason for that havoc was an overzealous application of a screening technology to a group of women for whom there was no scientific proof that the technology was beneficial.

DIAGNOSIS

Technologic advances in medical diagnosis have boomed in only a couple of decades. But they did not always find ready acceptance. Computed tomographic (CT) scanning was resisted vigorously. It was resisted for the same reasons, almost, that the stethoscope was resisted by the *London Times*. There was an irrational concern about whether this expensive piece of equipment really should be let loose. Now, of course, CT scanning has replaced less accurate procedures that are more costly and dangerous. It has been improved in use and it has become an adjunct to other diagnostic technologies and therapeutic technologies. It has done almost anything you could ask of a technology and has reduced cost and suffering to an enormous degree. Reduction in suffering is very hard to calculate in economic terms but is real to patients nonetheless. We are about to replay the CT story on a newer imaging technology. The subject this time is magnetic resonance imaging (MRI). This is a technology of high initial expense that is able to give tremendously accurate information about selected areas of the human anatomy and selected disorders. It needs a period of time during which people can learn to use it and learn and apply the possibilities it affords. Then we can begin to ask the rigorous questions required before the wider diffusion of MRI.

That is the positive side on diagnosis. What is the negative side? Endoscopy offers perhaps the best example. Fiber-optic endoscopy came forward with great promise. The assumption was that without using radiation one could look inside a patient and see, for example, upper gastrointestinal bleeding, discern the site of the bleeding, treat the patient more specifically, and improve the survival rate.

Everything happened except the last. The survival rate for upper intestinal bleeding is exactly what it has been for the past 25 years. And yet there is an increasing use of endoscopy in patients with gastrointestinal bleeding, even though the scientific foundation for its effect on outcome is weak. The continued application of a test on the basis of an unsubstantiated rationale does not help the introduction and diffusion of technology.

My general observation is that when we have introduced better methods of diagnosis to improve patient outcome the improvement has rarely occurred. Better diagnosis probably has helped to discern the natural history of disease, but better outcomes have generally resulted from better insights into the mechanism of disease. That is not to say that more accurate diagnosis should be eschewed. It is to say that the real reason for better methods of diagnosis seldom is that treatment will suddenly be more effective.

THERAPY

Turning to the subject of therapy, we also have subsets. We can classify it into Lewis Thomas's "supportive therapy," "halfway technology," and really effective "high technology." Supportive means that there is no therapy to be offered. It is illustrated in the old Luke Fildes painting of the doctor sitting at a child's bedside, worrying terribly about the patient but having no therapeutic skills. Under those circumstances, supportive care was all that could be offered. I am not suggesting that comforting a patient is unimportant. It is obviously very important; it simply is not as effective as proven medical or surgical therapy most of the time and also it is an exceedingly expensive use of resources for very little return.

So, we move to the next step, as described by Lewis Thomas.

At the next level up [after supportive therapy] is a kind of technology best termed "halfway technology." This represents the kinds of things that must be done after the fact, in efforts to compensate for the incapacitating effects of certain diseases whose course one is unable to do very much about. It is a technology designed to make up for disease or to postpone death.

The outstanding examples in recent years are transplantations of hearts, kidneys, livers, and other organs, and the equally spectacular inventions of artificial organs. In the public mind, this kind of technology has come to seem like the equivalent of the high technologies of the physical sciences. The media tend to present each new procedure as though it represented a breakthrough and a therapeutic triumph, instead of the makeshift that it really is.

In fact, this level of technology is, by its nature, at the same time highly sophisticated and profoundly primitive. It is the kind of thing that one must continue to do until there is genuine understanding of the mechanisms involved in disease. . . .

It is a characteristic of this kind of technology that it costs an enormous amount of money and requires a continuing expansion of hospital facilities. There is no end to the need for new, highly trained people to run the enterprise. And there is really no way out of this at the present state of knowledge. . . . The only thing that can move medicine away from this level of technology is new information, and the only imaginable source of this information is research (Thomas, 1974).

Thomas goes on to discuss the ideal technology, which includes a vaccine for preventing a disease, the replacement of an enzyme, the administration of a hormone to replace a deficiency state. These almost invariably inexpensive technological interventions turn out in the long run to be far more successful in maintaining or returning health.

Dr. Thomas makes the argument that investment in halfway technology is not worthwhile, and that the investment ought to be put into basic investigation. However, I see some problems with that approach. Take the instance of end-stage renal disease. Dialysis is available, and there is no question about what will happen to a person with renal failure if dialysis or transplantation is not provided. The person will die. The treatment is efficacious and the patient lives. The level of living ranges from those who can work to those who are incapacitated. The issue is not whether death from renal failure can be prevented. The issue is whether to expend the resources necessary to do that, and whether to encompass as broad a group of individuals as we are now treating.

The lithotriptor is an example of cost in the other direction. The lithotriptor is a machine that sends shock waves, focused from outside the body, into the body to converge at a kidney stone and gradually to hammer that stone into little pieces so that it can be passed. Thus, renal calculus removal has gone from a surgical incision with a six-week to two-month recovery period to a noninvasive procedure in which we can break up the stone 60 to 80 percent of the time in one day, and have the patient back at work in less than a week.

Yet, we are seeing the same sort of resistance to the lithotriptor that we have seen to every other major piece of technology. The machine does pose important questions. They have to do with whether we wish to allow a lithotriptor in every physician's office or whether we can regionalize it, given the relatively nonemergency circumstances for which it is used. Those issues concern policy, but to slow the lithotriptor's availability to individuals because we cannot deal with policy deprives people of the safest and most effective therapy— almost.

The best therapy is preventive. There is a broad group of patients with cystine, uric acid, and calcium stone diseases for whom medical therapy will reduce or prevent stone formations. This is where the conflict comes in. How much should be invested to provide individuals with a safety net (in the form of a lithotriptor) when that safety net also provides them with a reason not to follow their own programs in preventing illness? That conflict becomes a major concern in therapy and most obvious in the area of coronary artery disease, where the discussions have become convoluted.

In coronary artery disease, all of the approaches to its diagnosis and treatment could be reduced in their use if we practiced better preventive medicine. The content of prevention is gradually taking shape: the control of hypertension, the control of body weight, and the improvement of dietary habits. But if we took these preventive measures, the question would arise: Do we really need to become progressively more sophisticated in managing what will possibly be a smaller and smaller number of coronary disease patients? I do not have the answer, but that kind of question is emerging also as surgery is gradually being replaced in some patients by balloon angioplasty. Instead of opening the patient's chest, a balloon can be inserted through a peripheral artery and inflated to open the coronary vessels in 5 or 10 percent of coronary artery disease patients, and that rate of application will improve as the technique and technology get better.

One view is that angioplasty improvements will reduce costs dramatically for the procedure. The counteropinion is that lower cost per procedure will make it available to many more people and raise overall costs. If that latter argument holds, fallacious as it is, we might as well go out of business.

Perhaps one of the better examples of the conflict in technologic therapy is in the use of cardiac pacemakers. They are tremendously beneficial to patients, and yet they have been overused because the doctors do not always understand the indications and circumstances under which they should be used. They are, nonetheless, very effective. One patient who had a pacemaker put in looked up from his bed at a cardiac monitor and saw the pacer pacing and his heart following. He felt "a new, unwarranted but irrepressible kind of vanity."

I had come into the presence of a technological marvel, namely me. To be sure, the pacemaker is a wonderful miniature piece of high technology, my friend the surgeon a skilled worker in high technology, but the greatest of wonders is my own pump, my myocardium, capable of accepting electronic instructions from that small black box and doing exactly what it is told. I am exceedingly pleased with my machine-tooled, obedient, responsive self. I would never have thought I had it in me, but now that I have it in me, ticking along soundlessly, flawlessly, I am subject to waves of pure vanity. . . .

I suppose I should be feeling guilty about this. In a way I do, for I have written and lectured in the past about medicine's excessive dependence on technology in general, and the resultant escalation in the cost of health care. I have been critical of what I have called "halfway technologies," designed to shore things up and keep flawed organs functioning beyond their appointed time. And here I am, enjoying precisely this sort of technology, eating my words (Thomas, 1984).

That was also written by Lewis Thomas. The perspective of the patient, who benefits from the technology, versus the policymaker, who is trying to decide how it should be used, must be kept in mind.

REHABILITATION

I will address technologic advances in rehabilitation only briefly. We are approaching a time when neural transplantation may be possible or when the regeneration of nerves will be facilitated. These advances will be coupled with computer-assisted limbs. The opportunity to return people from a dependent status to a functional status is upon us, and I think we are going to have to take advantage of it. But again, the reimbursement structure does not yet recognize such technologic applications, and the same arguments will occur in dealing with highly expensive systems in the rehabilitative sector as are now occurring in pacemaker and cardiac surgical technology.

What should we as physicians do? My sense is that we should develop a framework for technological innovation with well-defined priorities, ranking prevention and screening higher than therapeutic interventions. That set of priorities could be developed in the framework that I have presented or almost any other, but physicians certainly should play a key role in the process. Safety and efficacy are important, but utility in the clinical setting must also be considered.

The way we use most medical devices in practice depends on postintroduction modifications of the devices. We work together—the physicians and the manufacturers and the engineers—in such modifications, and suggestions gradually get built into the device. Assessment of what we have accomplished becomes very important.

A broadly receptive system of information, which can be transferred to physicians and to patients, now is critical in the application of new technologies. The random input from consultant or journal or newspaper is no way to learn how new technology works. It is time to pay much more attention to the monitoring of new technology after it has been introduced. Such monitoring is easy to do in hospitals; it will be relatively easy in managed care systems. It may be difficult in the individual physician's office and abuses may occur there, but we have no excuse for not taking on all areas in which the system can be monitored and examined.

If these actions are seen not in terms of protecting the ability to develop a new device, nor in terms of protecting physicians and innovators from liability, but as selecting and evolving the most appropriate use for new technology in support of health, then I think we have a process that will bring together medicine, engineering, and industry in a very exciting enterprise.

REFERENCES

McKusick, V. A. 1958. Cardiovascular Sound in Health and Disease. Baltimore: Williams & Wilkins.

Thier, S. O. 1983. Pp. xiii–xiv *in* Laboratory Medicine in Clinical Practice, Harvey N. Mandell, ed. Boston: John Wright PSG, Inc.

Thomas, L. 1974. The technology of medicine. Pp. 31–36 *in* The Lives of a Cell: Notes of a Biology Watcher. New York: Viking.

Thomas, L. 1984. My magical metronome. Pp. 45–48 *in* Late Night Thoughts on Listening to Mahler's Ninth Symphony. New York: Bantam Books.

Inventing Medical Devices: Five Inventors' Stories

Development of Technicon's Auto Analyzer

EDWIN C. WHITEHEAD

In 1950 Alan Moritz, chairman of the department of pathology at Case Western Reserve University and an old friend of mine, wrote to tell me about Leonard Skeggs, a young man in his department who had developed an instrument that Technicon might be interested in. I was out of my New York office on a prolonged trip, and my father, cofounder with me of Technicon Corporation, opened the letter. He wrote to Dr. Moritz saying that Technicon was always interested in new developments and enclosed a four-page confidential disclosure form. Not surprisingly, Dr. Moritz thought that Technicon was not really interested in Skeggs's instrument, and my father dismissed the matter as routine.

Three years later Ray Roesch, Technicon's only salesman at the time, was visiting Joseph Kahn at the Cleveland Veterans Administration Hospital. Dr. Kahn asked Ray why Technicon had turned down Skeggs's invention. Ray responded that he had never heard of it and asked, "What invention?" Kahn replied, "A machine to automate chemical analysis." When Ray called me and asked why I had turned Skeggs's idea down, I said I had not heard of it either. When he told me that Skeggs's idea was to automate clinical chemistry, my reaction was, "Wow! Let's look at it and make sure Skeggs doesn't get away."

That weekend, Ray Roesch loaded some laboratory equipment in his station wagon and drove Leonard Skeggs and his wife Jean to New York. At Technicon, Skeggs set up a simple device consisting of a peristaltic pump to draw the specimen sample and reagent streams through the system, a continuous dialyzer to remove protein molecules

13

that might interfere with the specimen-reagent reaction, and a spectrophotometer equipped with a flow cell to monitor the reaction. This device demonstrated the validity of the idea, and we promptly entered negotiations with Skeggs for a license to patent the Auto Analyzer. We agreed on an initial payment of $6,000 and royalties of 3 percent after a certain number of units had been sold.

After Technicon "turned-down" the project in 1950, Skeggs had made arrangements first with the Heinecke Instrument Co. and then the Harshaw Chemical Co. to sell his device. Both companies erroneously assumed that the instrument was a finished product. However, neither company had been able to sell a single instrument from 1950 until 1953. This was not surprising, because Skeggs's original instrument required an expensive development process to make it rugged and reliable, and to modify the original, manual chemical assays. Technicon spent 3 years refining the simple model developed by Skeggs into a commercially viable continuous-flow analyzer.

A number of problems unique to the Auto Analyzer had to be overcome. Because the analyzer pumps a continuous-flow stream of reagents interrupted by specimen samples, one basic problem was the interaction between specimen samples. This problem was alleviated by introducing air bubbles as physical barriers between samples. However, specimen carryover in continuous-flow analyzers remains sensitive to the formation and size of bubbles, the inside diameter of the tubing through which fluids flow, the pattern of peristaltic pumping action, and other factors.

Development of the Auto Analyzer was financed internally at Technicon. In 1953 Technicon had ongoing business of less than $10 million per year: automatic tissue processors and slide filing cabinets for histology laboratories, automatic fraction collectors for chromatography, and portable respirators for polio patients. Until it went public in 1969, Technicon had neither borrowed money nor sold equity. Thus, Technicon's patent on Skeggs's original invention was central to the development of the Auto Analyzer. Without patent protection, Technicon could never have afforded to pursue the expensive development of this device.

Early in the instrument's development, I recognized that traditional marketing techniques suitable for most laboratory instruments would not work for something as revolutionary as the Auto Analyzer. At that time, laboratory instruments were usually sold by catalog salesmen or by mail from specification sheets listing instrument specifications, price, and perhaps product benefits. In contrast, we decided that

Technicon had to market the Auto Analyzer as a complete system— instrument, reagents, and instruction.

Technicon's marketing strategy has been to promote the Auto Analyzer at professional meetings and through scientific papers and journal articles. Technicon employs only direct salesmen. The company has never used agents or distributors, except in countries where the market is too small to support direct sales.

To introduce technology as radical as the Auto Analyzer into conservative clinical laboratories, Technicon decided to perform clinical evaluations. Although unusual at that time, such evaluations have since become commonplace. An important condition of the clinical evaluations was Technicon's insistence that the laboratory conducting the evaluation call a meeting of its local professional society to announce the results. Such meetings generally resulted in an enthusiastic endorsement of the Auto Analyzer by the laboratory director. I believe this technique had much to do with the rapid market acceptance of the Auto Analyzer.

Other unusual marketing strategies employed by Technicon to promote the Auto Analyzer included symposia and training courses. Technicon sponsored about 25 symposia on techniques in automated analytical chemistry. The symposia were generally 3-day affairs, attracting between 1,000 and 4,500 scientists, and were held in most of the major countries of the world including the United States.

Because we realized that market acceptance of the Auto Analyzer could be irreparably damaged by incompetent users, Technicon set up a broad-scale training program. We insisted that purchasers of Auto Analyzers come to our training centers located around the world for a 1-week course of instruction. I estimate that we have trained about 50,000 people to use Auto Analyzers.

Introduction of Technicon's continuous-flow Auto Analyzer in 1957 profoundly changed the character of the clinical laboratory, allowing a hundredfold increase in the number of laboratory tests performed over a 10-year period. When we began to develop the Auto Analyzer in 1953, I estimated a potential market of 250 units. Currently, more than 50,000 Auto Analyzer Channels are estimated to be in use around the world.

In reviewing the 35-year history of the Auto Analyzer, I have come to the conclusion that several factors significantly influenced our success. First, the Auto Analyzer allowed both an enormous improvement in the quality of laboratory test results and an enormous reduction in the cost of doing chemical analysis. Second, physicians began to realize that accurate laboratory data are useful in diagnosis. Last, reimbursement policies increased the availability of health care.

Plasmapheresis

EDWIN C. WHITEHEAD

In the early 1940s, I read a provocative article by Arthur Wright, professor of surgery at New York University. Dr. Wright observed that by removing the plasma from a blood donation and then reinfusing red blood cells in the donor, one could bleed the donor twice a week instead of once every 7 weeks.

At the time, Technicon Corporation was doing some work with William Aaronson, who was a pathologist at Morrisania Hospital in New York and also had a private laboratory. He and I discussed Wright's article and decided that the process would be practical only if it were automated. Otherwise, taking a blood donation, separating the cells from the plasma, and reinfusing the red blood cells in the donor would be too laborious.

This was during World War II, and every newspaper and advertisement called for donations of plasma, which was sorely needed by the military. Dr. Aaronson and I reasoned that, since most of the soldiers in the United States were young and healthy, bleeding soldiers twice a week might be a better way of obtaining plasma than depending on donations from the civilian population. If we could make a small, portable, rugged, relatively inexpensive device to automate the process described by Wright, the military and the Red Cross should have great need for it.

Aaronson and I experimented to determine the most efficient way to separate blood and plasma. The design we finally settled on was a cone-shaped container with radially extending blades that divided the container into separate compartments. Blood was drawn from the donor through a needle and injected directly into the center of the spinning container. Red cells were packed by centrifugal force at the outer edges of the container and plasma formed a layer closer to the center. We started removing plasma as soon as we had drawn 100 ml of blood. By the time the 400-ml blood donation was drawn, the plasma had been removed into a plastic bag. Saline solution was then added to the donor's red blood cells and the cells were fed back to the donor by gravity through the same needle used to draw the blood.

In 6 months we had developed an operating prototype. We decided to try it out by hiring a professional blood donor, bleeding the donor twice a week, and doing weekly blood chemistry studies to see if the donor experienced any ill effects. We managed to find a donor, but when we explained what we intended to do, he looked first startled, then frightened, and quickly picked up his hat and walked out.

Aaronson and I tried to enlist other paid donors with the same result and finally decided to test our prototype by bleeding each other. I would stop at Aaronson's laboratory on my way home from work each Monday and Friday afternoon, and we would bleed each other. In 1944, after 6 months of observing no adverse effects, we decided that it was time to market the device.

We made appointments with Red Cross, Army, and Navy offices in Washington, D.C., to demonstrate the device. Aaronson and I boarded the train from New York to Washington carrying a large box that contained substantial quantities of donated whole blood packed in ice. Feeling pleased with ourselves, we had reserved seats in the club car. We plunked down our large box and took our seats. Near Philadelphia, we noticed a thin, red stream of blood running from the box. Although our fellow passengers were too polite to comment, we were so embarrassed that we pretended the box did not belong to us until we got to Washington. Fortunately, only one of the bottles had broken.

When Aaronson and I arrived in Washington, we were told by the Red Cross, the Army, and the Navy that, despite public appeals, the one thing the military had in abundance was blood plasma! In fact, both the Navy and the Army made a point of telling us that the first thing to be jettisoned in time of battle was blood plasma. Thus, our "market" completely disappeared and we abandoned our project, having spent a considerable amount of effort and receiving a patent for our invention.

Pneumatic Extradural
Intracranial Pressure Monitor

ALAN R. KAHN

Intracranial pressure (ICP) is monitored to detect dangerous pressure increases in patients with head or spinal trauma, craniotomies, Reye's syndrome, and certain drug intoxications. Before the invention of the pneumatic extradural ICP monitor in 1980, monitoring of ICP was generally accomplished by means of fluid-filled catheters (or other similar appliances) with one end in direct contact with the patient's cerebrospinal fluid and the other end connected to a conventional pressure transducer. A device that detects ICP from a site outside the dura (the outermost and toughest membrane covering the brain) had been on the market for several years, but the pressure sensor in that device is very complicated and fragile, is slow to respond to changes, and is limited in accuracy. Thus, although that device established the usefulness of extradural ICP monitoring and has found application in certain medical centers, its use has been limited because of the complexity and inaccuracy of its sensing system.

In contrast, the pneumatic extradural ICP monitoring system makes it possible to measure ICP simply, accurately, and at low cost. The invention includes a disposable sensor that is accurate, rugged, and inexpensive to construct. The invention also includes a pneumatic system in a monitoring module that powers the sensor and provides self-checking and failure detection. The system has been designed as a sophisticated microprocessor-based instrument and has been introduced to the market by Meadox Instruments, Inc.

THE INVENTION PROCESS

The invention of the ICP monitor was not the result of new technological developments but was rather the application of a basic physical principle that had been overlooked in the area of pressure measurement. In recent years, advances in technology have been made primarily in the field of electronics, and scientists and engineers tend to ignore other physical modalities such as pneumatics. Most of my inventions have been in the area of sensing and measurement and make use of basic physics rather than new technological developments. The necessary technical information can be found in any basic physics textbook.

I first had the idea for the pressure management technique used in this instrument in 1964 as a way to measure the elasticity of human skin for a study on aging. At the time, I worked for a major corporation that did not see a market for a device with that application, and no product was ever developed.

In 1980, during a discussion on ICP monitoring, I realized that my old idea could be modified for use in this new application. I offered the company with which I was employed the opportunity to develop this product under a royalty arrangement, but the company declined. Subsequently, I left that company to join a research and development consulting firm as an equal partner with the two existing partners, and we invested our time and personal funds to develop a prototype ICP monitoring system. It took 6 months to build and test the first prototype in our laboratory and to perform preliminary tests in animals.

FINANCING AND MARKETING

Perhaps the most difficult step we encountered was in obtaining funding for design and marketing of the product. This was complicated by the fact that my partners and I were primarily interested in the R&D process and did not wish to get involved in marketing. Negotiations with venture capital firms and other conventional sources of capital proved unsuccessful, because acceptance of the extradural method of ICP monitoring was limited by the existing product, and it was difficult to project just how an improved product would affect market growth. Therefore, conservative sales projections were used in the business plan. These projections made the venture less attractive and affected our ability to obtain funding.

We finally established a joint venture with Meadox, a biomedical company that had facilities for manufacturing the sensors and saw our ICP monitoring device as an efficient way to enter the market for electronic products. Each of the three partners in our R&D firm owned 9 percent of the new joint venture company and shared a royalty on product sales. Our R&D company received a contract from the joint venture company to develop the product and subsequently to manufacture the electronic portion of the system until such time as the contractors learned more about the product and could take over all of the manufacturing. Although sales of the ICP monitoring systems in the United States proceeded as anticipated in our conservative projection, the monitoring device was foreign to the Meadox product line and was subsequently discontinued.

Invention of an Electronic Retinoscope

ARAN SAFIR

Following a year at Cornell University as an engineering student, I entered the U.S. Navy when I turned 18. On the basis of an aptitude test, I was placed in a training program for electronic technicians. The training lasted nearly a year and was rigorous and thorough. My Navy training and World War II ended almost simultaneously, and I spent another year in the Navy working on aircraft radio and radar systems.

During that year, I decided that a career in medicine might offer a good combination of science, technology, and the social disciplines. I entered New York University as a premedical student majoring in English; later I entered medical school. Medical school was not much fun—rote memorization is not my strongest skill. In retrospect, I can see the early indications of some factors that would later assume great importance in my life.

In high school, I had been seriously interested in photography—both the technology and the art. I had neither time nor money for it in medical school, but I turned to optics to help me learn pathology. Each student was given hundreds of slides of pathology specimens to be studied under the microscope so that the features of various diseases could be memorized. While studying my slides, I discovered that I could place my microscope on the floor underneath a small table that had a ground glass top. When I darkened the room, I could see the projected image of the microscope slide on the tabletop.

Thus, I set about making my microscope into a projector. I bought the most powerful truck headlight bulb I could find, attached it to a transformer through an adjustable resistor so that I could operate the bulb well above its rated voltage, purchased some surplus lenses, and soldered together various rectangular and cylindrical tin cans to form a powerful substage lamp for my microscope. A small prism deflected the beam onto a white poster board on the wall, giving an image about 2 feet in diameter. With this device, several friends and I often studied our slides together and helped each other to learn.

Still, I thought of this as only a passing diversion, almost occupational therapy, because I had always been a good mechanic and enjoyed building things. About 2 years later, I had a brief exposure to ophthalmology, which is all that most medical students get. But even during that brief exposure, I realized that I had to make almost no effort to memorize those parts of the textbook that dealt with the formation of images by the eye. When we went to the ophthalmological clinics and could look into the eyes of patients through widely dilated pupils, I was thrilled by the magic of the eye as an optical instrument.

It was not until many months later, during my internship, that I had any opportunity to try my hand at surgery. When I found that I was good at surgery and enjoyed it, I began to think seriously of ophthalmology as a career. Still, it was my intention at the time to become a practitioner of ophthalmology and to return to my hometown to establish a private practice. I clearly recall that at my residency interview at the New York Eye and Ear Infirmary, when the governing board of six senior surgeons asked me whether I intended to do research, my reply was: "I don't know. I think I would like to try, to see whether I'm any good at it."

I became a resident at the New York Eye and Ear Infirmary in 1956. That institution was known mostly for the excellent opportunity it gave the trainee to observe, learn, and participate in the practice of ophthalmology, but offered little experience or opportunity in research. There was a small scientific program, but residents were rarely involved.

I reported for duty as a resident at the infirmary on July 1, 1956. After being issued white uniforms, I was shown to the clinic. There I was put in the care of a second-year resident who was clearly too busy with his own clinical problems to spend much time with me. He sat me down on a stool in a little booth where a patient sat next to a box of ophthalmological trial lenses. This was to be my first experience with refraction of the eye. Handing me a small instrument that resembled a flashlight, which he told me was a retinoscope, the second-year resident explained that I was to look through the little hole in the mirror and direct the beam of light into the patient's pupil. When I shined the light into the patient's eye, he explained, I would observe the patient's pupil glowing with light reflected from inside the eye. By tilting the mirror, I could make the reflected light move across the pupil. I was to sit at arm's length from the patient and observe whether the light coming back out of the pupil moved in the same direction as the light I shined on the patient's face, or in the opposite direction. If the light moved in the same direction, I was to take lenses from one side of the box, while if the light moved in a contrary direction, I was to take them from the other side of the box. I was to select lenses that would make the light appear to stop moving. Wishing me good luck, the resident went off to his own tasks.

I worked very hard at this first refraction and was quite upset by it. Like other young physicians, I had spent years learning to be competent in difficult matters. To be thrust suddenly back into complete incompetence and at the same time to have responsibility for patient care was disturbing to me. I recall going to lunch that day and sitting across the table from that same second-year resident. I told him, "If I can see those lights moving in the pupil, I'll bet I can make a photoelectric device that will see them better and faster." That was the conception of my idea of an automatic retinoscope.

The retinoscope is basically a small lamp that shines light on a mirror with a hole in its center. Light reflected from the mirror enters the patient's pupil and illuminates the retina at the back of the eye. Nearly all the light is then absorbed, but a small fraction is reflected back, passes through the pupil, and leaves the patient's eye. The light that is reflected by the retina goes through the optical system of the patient's eye and acquires characteristics of that system.

The light rays leaving the eye can be either convergent, parallel, or divergent. If a patient's eye has excessive converging power, as it does in myopia (nearsightedness), the light rays leaving the eye will converge to a point in space at some distance in front of the eye. The distance from the patient's eye to that point is a measure of the amount of myopia (the closer the point to the eye, the greater the degree of myopia). An eye with no refractive error sends out parallel rays, and a farsighted eye sends out divergent rays.

The retinoscopist sits in front of the patient, looks through the sight hole in the center of the mirror, and decides whether the emerging light rays have reached a convergent point between him and the patient or have not yet converged by the time they get to his eye. The patient, merely has to hold fairly still and gaze at a distant target. The examiner puts lenses in front of the patient's eye to bring the convergent point to a standard place, at the examiner's eye. The lenses needed to accomplish this are a measure of the eye's refractive state.

With this objective measurement, the examiner can go to the next phase of the examination, in which the patient's subjective responses to various lenses are elicited. There is usually good agreement between retinoscopic measurements and the patient's subjective responses. Because retinoscopy depends on the examiner's skill, which varies considerably among practitioners, and the patient's subjective responses, are affected by the patient's personality, the final judgment of the patient's visual status often requires complex decision making.

Shortly after beginning my work in the clinic, I drew up plans for the construction of an electronic retinoscope and presented my ideas to the research committee of the New York Eye and Ear Infirmary. I asked them for sufficient laboratory space and a budget for some equipment so that I might try out my idea. They gave me about 6 feet of bench space in someone else's laboratory, allowed me to borrow a double-beam oscilloscope, and gave me a drawing account of about $500. I set to work building an instrument.

The hospital had a lathe and a drill press that were gathering dust for want of a machine shop, so I was asked to build one for them. With the aid of one of the hospital's engineering staff, I constructed a machine shop to which I was subsequently given free access.

The chief administrator of the hospital recommended that I obtain a patent on my invention and suggested that I go to a former West Point classmate of his who had become a senior partner in a well-known New York patent firm. I did this, and the senior patent attorney assigned my case to a young patent attorney who had just joined the firm. That was when I found out that patent attorneys have degrees both in law and in a scientific discipline. In the young attorney's case, it was electrical engineering.

The New York Eye and Ear Infirmary gave me a key to the library and research building and, over the course of about a year and with the aid of my attorney friend, I built a working model of the electronic retinoscope. The instrument was crude—the photocells were housed in the film carrier of an old view camera, the image of the subject eye was formed by a telescope made from the mailing tube that had held my diploma from medical school, and many of the parts were surplus that I had purchased at the outdoor hardware stalls on Canal Street in New York. But 18 months after I started, I had a working model that demonstrated the feasibility of the method and was able to measure the refractive state of schematic eyes, which are metal and glass simulations of human eyes and are commercially available to students of refraction who are learning retinoscopy.

An important scene stands out in my memory of those times. As soon as the retinoscope was operating satisfactorily, I invited a few close friends to come and see it. Rather late one evening we gathered in the lab: my patent attorney, my girlfriend, and three or four ophthalmological buddies. I explained the device and what to look for on the oscilloscope, dimmed the room lights, and put the instrument through its paces. The outputs of the photocells could be easily seen on the oscilloscope. As the schematic eye was changed from nearsighted to farsighted, the oscilloscope tracing showed the change and clearly identified the crucial neutral point when the convergent point of the rays emerging from the eye was brought to precisely the correct distance, exactly as in clinical retinoscopy.

The instrument had a rotating light beam deflector for creating the scan of light across the eye. There were mirrors and lenses that cast moving patterns of light, not only on the schematic eye, but on the walls of the lab as well. The oscilloscope face flickered with green evanescent tracings. In the darkened lab, it was dramatic.

As others got interested in the apparatus and began to operate it themselves, I stepped back to the far side of the room and watched them. A new feeling swept over me and I verbalized it internally: "Look at what I have done. What started as an idea in my head has created a new machine and has gathered these people here and captured their interest." I had a feeling of power and wonder, a very good feeling, and though I have experienced it again since then, it has never been so poignant. Surely, there are many reasons for people to experience such feelings, but invention is one that I have known, and I suspect that those who do not invent do not often appreciate the emotional importance of the act.

The young patent attorney was rather excited about this project because his review of the patents in existence had led him to conclude that we were opening up an entirely new field. The idea of dynamic scanning to measure an optical system had not been patented before. After about 2 years of effort, we filed a patent application in 1958. The patent was not granted until 1964, after several rejections and a hearing. The entire 6-year proceeding, which cost me a great deal of money and effort, seemed to be designed to test my persistence rather than my inventiveness.

In 1964 I received a letter from Bausch & Lomb asking me if I was interested in licensing my patent to them. A contractual agreement was arranged between the Bausch & Lomb Company and me. It was 8 years from the time we signed the contract until Bausch & Lomb offered an instrument for sale. In that time, another company came out with an automatic refracting machine, and the Bausch & Lomb retinoscope never achieved a significant share of the market. Now there are several automatic refracting machines on the market. Most of them are made in Japan, and one of them made by a major Japanese company uses the principle that I patented. For this, the company paid me royalties during the last year of the life of my patent.

I made very little money from this invention. If I were to reckon my income from it in dollars earned per hours spent, I would have been far better off to have spent my time practicing ophthalmology.

The First Successful Implantable Cardiac Pacemaker

WILSON GREATBATCH

On April 7, 1958 Dr. William C. Chardack, Dr. Andrew Gage, and I implanted the first self-powered implantable cardiac pacemaker in an experimental animal. In October of that year, Dr. Ake Senning in Stockholm attempted the first human implant. That device worked for only 3 hours and then failed. A replacement device worked for 8 days, after which the patient survived unstimulated for 3 years. Two years later, in 1960, Dr. Chardack, Dr. Gage, and I implanted the first successful cardiac pacemaker in a human.

At the time, we predicted an annual use of perhaps 10,000 pacemakers per year. Soon thereafter, however, the implantable pacemaker became the treatment of choice for complete heart block (impairment of conduction in heart excitation) with Stokes-Adams syndrome (a condition caused by heart block and characterized by sudden attacks of unconsciousness). Today—nearly 30 years later—pacemakers have assumed forms and functions that we never dreamed of, and the world pacemaker market is approaching 300,000 units per year.

When World War II was over in 1945, I decided to register at the School of Electrical Engineering at Cornell University in Ithaca, New York. As an undergraduate at Cornell, I got my first exposure to medical electronics. To feed my family, I occasionally worked as an electronics technician, building intermediate-frequency amplifiers for what was later to become the Arecibo, Puerto Rico, radiotelescope. One day, in an adjacent lab, I saw Cornell graduate student Frank Noble measuring blood pressure in a rat by recording the change in tail size as a pulse of blood traversed it. Frank's electronic plethysmograph belonged to the psychology department's Animal Behavior Farm at Varna, New York, near Ithaca. Research at the Animal Behavior Farm dealt with conditioned reflex under neurosis, and Frank was responsible for measuring heart rate and blood pressure in some 100 sheep and goats there. I became very interested in this work, and when Frank left to become head of an electronics laboratory at the National Institutes of Health, I inherited his job.

During the summer of 1951, two New England brain surgeons spent their summer sabbatical at the farm performing experimental brain surgery on the hypothalamus of goats. At lunchtime we would sit on the grass in the bright Ithaca sun and talk shop. I learned much practical physiology during our discussions. One day, the subject of heart block came up. When the surgeons described it, I knew I could fix it—but not with the vacuum tubes and storage batteries then available.

By the time the first commercial silicon transistors became available (at $90 each) in 1956, I had become an assistant professor of electrical engineering at the University of Buffalo, I was also spending time with Dr. Simon Rodbard and Dr. Robert Cohn at the Chronic Disease Research Institute in Buffalo.

Sy Rodbard was interested in fast heart sounds, which we recorded with an oscilloscope and a movie camera. I wanted a 1-kilohertz marker oscillator and built one out of a single transistor and a United Transformer Company model DOT–1 (UTC DOT–1) transformer. My marker oscillator used a 10-kilohm base-bias resistor. One day, I reached into my resistor box to get a 10-kilohm resistor but misread the color codes, and instead of getting the brown-black-orange resistor, I got a brown-black-green (1 megohm) resistor. The circuit started to squeg (oscillate in bursts) with a 1.8-millisecond pulse followed by a 1-second quiescent interval. During the quiescent interval, the transistor was cut off and drew practically no current. I stared at the thing in disbelief and then realized that this was *exactly* what was needed to drive a heart. I built a few more. For the next 5 years, most of the world's pacemakers were to use a blocking oscillator with a UTC DOT-1 transformer just because I grabbed the wrong resistor!

I found little enthusiasm locally for an implantable cardiac pacemaker. Each medical group I approached said, "Fine idea, but most of these patients die in a year or so. Why don't you work on my project?"

In Buffalo we had the first local chapter in the world of the Institute of Radio Engineers, Professional Group in Medical Electronics (the IRE/PGME, now the Biomedical Engineering Society of the Institute of Electrical and Electronics Engineers). Every month, 25 to 75 doctors and engineers met for a technical program. Our chapter had a standing offer to send an engineering team to assist any doctor who had an instrumentation problem. One day in the spring of 1958, I went with such a team to visit Dr. William Chardack on a problem dealing with a blood oximeter. Dr. Chardack was Chief of Surgery at the Veterans Administration Hospital in Buffalo. Imagine my surprise at finding that his assistant was one of my old high school classmates, Andy Gage (later chief of staff at the hospital)! Our visiting team could not help Dr. Chardack much with his blood oximeter problem, but when I broached my pacemaker idea to him, he walked up and down the lab a couple of times, looked at me strangely, and said, "If you can do that, you can save 10,000 lives a year." Three weeks later in April 1958, Dr. Chardack, Dr. Gage, and I had our first model cardiac pacemaker implanted in a dog.

Our experimental work was done on dogs that had been put into complete heart block by occluding the atrioventricular (AV) bundle with a tied suture. We had no heart-lung machine. The operating team stood poised like runners waiting for the starting gun. Upon a "go" signal, the team occluded the large vessels, opened the heart, occluded the AV bundle with the tied suture, closed the heart, and released the large vessels, all in 90 seconds!

We were naive about early pacemaker designs. We initially thought that wrapping the module in electric tape would seal it. We soon found, however, that any void beneath the tape would fill with fluid, so we began to case our electronics in a solid epoxy block. Within a year, we had worked our animal survival time up from 4 hours to 4 months and felt ready to start looking for a suitable patient.

Building pacemaker units began taking more of my time than my job would allow, so I quit my job to work full time on the pacemaker in 1960. I had $2,000 in cash and enough to feed my family for 2 years. I took the $2,000 and went up into my wood-heated barn workshop. In 2 years I had made 50 pacemakers, 40 of which went into animals and 10 into patients.

The 10 patients had their pacemakers implanted by Dr. Chardack and his associates. Most of the patients were older people in their sixties, seventies, and eighties, typical of the usual heart-block patient. However, two of the patients were children and one was a young man with a wife and two children. The young man, I remember, had worked in a local rubber factory until he collapsed on the job one day. Soon thereafter, he had another severe attack in which his mother-in-law applied resuscitation and brought him back. Before implantation of the pacemaker, the young man's prognosis was grim. After recovery, he retrained as a hairdresser, worked full time, and joined a bowling team. This man was still alive and well in late 1987. Another patient I remember well, also in complete heart block with Stokes-Adams syndrome, was a woman in her sixties. She was our seventh patient. A few years ago, when our local engineering society named me "Engineer of the Year," she came to my award dinner. The news media called her the "Pacemaker Queen." She died not too long ago, in her eighties, after having been paced for over 20 years.

In early 1961, Jim Anderson and Palmer Hermundslie of the Medtronic Company, which manufactured external, hand-held pacemakers, flew into Buffalo from Minneapolis. At a luncheon table in the Airways Hotel at the Buffalo airport, we worked out a license agreement for the implantable cardiac pacemaker. The next day we had it notarized at a local bank. This agreement was the beginning of the Medtronic Chardack-Greatbatch Implantable Cardiac Pacemaker, which dominated the field for the next decade.

The license agreement was a very tight one. I assumed design control for all Medtronic implantable pacemakers. I signed every drawing, every change, and had to approve every procurement source. The device had to be called a "Chardack-Greatbatch Implantable Cardiac Pacemaker" in all company brochures, advertising, and communications, both within the company and without. The quality control program reported directly to me for 10 years. I sat on the board of directors and had a major (and noisy) input to all company affairs, pushing pacemakers and dropping unprofitable product lines like cardiac monitors and defibrillators. Within 2 years Medtronic had become number one in pacemakers. Today, over two decades later, Medtronic is still number one, and has a sales volume of nearly $300 million a year.

Dr. Chardack was just as active as I, but in an unofficial, behind-the-scenes way. His papers, his case reports, his spring-coil electrodes, and his personal recommendations really "sold" the Medtronic device to the profession. Dr. Chardack's professional stature and reputation in the field were unparalleled. He was Medtronic's most effective and most credible "salesman" in those critical early days.

We soon found that the highest grade military components were not good enough for the "zero defect" requirements of pacemakers. The warm, moist environment of the human body proved to be a far more hostile environment than outer space or the bottom of the sea. We had predicted a 5-year pacemaker in our first 1959 paper, but even by 1970 we were getting only 2 years.

The miniature DOT–1 transformers that we initially used were wound with exceptionally fine wire and proved troublesome. We continued to experience failures until we finally went to a transformerless design. The Medtronic 5862 (my last design for Medtronic) used a three-transistor, transformerless, complementary multivibrator circuit (after Roger Russell's patent) which could not "hang up." With diode-isolated, dual-battery packs and voltage-doubler output, it was probably the most reliable of the mercury-powered pacemakers of the 1960s.

Early transistors were inconsistent. We identified several failure modes due to contamination and leaky seals. We adopted the policy of segregating the transistors into beta (current gain) classes and then heat-soaking them for 500 hours at 125°C; they were transferred to dry ice five times during this period. Any transistor that developed leakage or drifted more than one beta class was discarded. This was followed by a shock test. We lost about 15 percent of the GE 2N335 transistors in this program, but never lost one subsequently in a pacemaker. (The Minuteman space program later adopted much the same approach for high-reliability missile components after we published our procedures.)

In 1964 Barough Berkovits (also a member of our chapter of the Professional Group in Medical Electronics when the American Optical Company Medical Electronics Division was in Buffalo) published a series of papers on a new pacemaker concept in which the pacemaker "listened" to the heart and worked only when the heart did not. A "demand pacemaker" seemed like quite a good idea, and we began working on an implantable version. My laboratory notebook says that we completed our first successful prototype on January 10, 1965. This design went on to become the Medtronic model 5841, which was the first implantable, inhibited-demand pacemaker to become commercially available.

We gradually improved pacemaker reliability to the point that battery quality became the limiting factor. It was increasingly apparent that we would never achieve our objective of a "lifetime pacemaker" with the zinc-mercury battery. I terminated my license with Medtronic under friendly circumstances and established my own battery manufacturing company, Wilson Greatbatch Ltd. Battery manufacturing, by the way, was another field about which I knew nothing.

By 1972, after looking into several types of batteries, we had settled on a battery with a lithium anode, an iodine cathode, and a solid-state, self-healing, crystalline electrolyte invented originally by Catalyst Research Corporation in Baltimore. The development of the lithium battery eventually removed the battery as the limiting factor in pacemaker longevity. Today, nearly every pacemaker uses a lithium battery of some sort, and nearly every surgical intervention for a pacemaker problem is electrode-related rather than battery-related.

Wheelchairs for the Third World

RALF HOTCHKISS

For the past 20 years I have been involved in wheelchair design and innovation. I became a paraplegic in 1966 and began by modifying my first chair. I now work full time on wheelchair design. For the past 12 years, I have been involved in making stair-climbing wheelchairs, stand/squat models, and high-speed sports chairs. My current focus is the design of lightweight folding wheelchairs for manufacture in developing countries.

NICARAGUA WHEELCHAIR PROJECT

In 1980 I was contacted by Bruce Curtis, a disabled man involved with the independent living movement. He had just returned from a trip to Caribbean and Central American countries, including Nicaragua. He was most enthusiastic about a group of disabled people he had met at a rehabilitation center in Managua, many of whom had become disabled during the revolution of 1979. These disabled Nicaraguans needed assistance with wheelchair repairs and wanted to learn to drive automobiles with hand controls. More important, they were very interested in the concept of independent living, which had given birth to numerous independent living centers in the United States.

On my first trip to Nicaragua in 1980, I met many disabled people and began to assess their problems in obtaining and maintaining affordable wheelchairs that would meet their needs. I found that the disabled Nicaraguans who had managed to get wheelchairs used two types of chairs. The vast majority of people had second- or third-hand hospital-type chairs, which had hard tires and nonremovable armrests and footrests, and which gave the users little flexibility of use or mobility. Such wheelchairs had frequent breakdowns and were not very useful outdoors. The second type of chair was a U.S. prescription model, which few people had because it was very expensive by Nicaraguan standards. This type of chair was easier to use but had many of the same problems as the others. It was heavy, and the seat widths of the standard imported models tended to be far too wide for Nicaraguans. Many common replacement parts were impossible to get because American wheelchairs are not made from generic, interchangeable parts.

During my 1980 trip, I also worked with disabled people from the United States to provide information to disabled Nicaraguans about independent living. This visit set into motion the formation of an independent living center organized and run by disabled Nicaraguans from the rehabilitation center. The Nicaraguan government gave the group a house in Managua to use as an office. One of the group's top priorities was to set up a wheelchair repair shop and to obtain new wheelchairs that Nicaraguans could afford. The group also began to plan for the eventual economic self-sufficiency of the independent living center.

After returning to the United States, I submitted a proposal to a Washington, D.C.-based group, Appropriate Technology International, which would allow me to provide technical assistance to the Managua independent living center for the establishment of a wheelchair repair and manufacturing shop. This proposal was funded for 1 year. During that year, I developed a prototype of a Third World-appropriate wheelchair at my shop in Oakland, California, and made eight trips to Nicaragua to help the independent living center organize its shop, purchase its tools and equipment, develop wheelchair repair and modification techniques, and begin making wheelchairs. Under a second contract with Appropriate Technology International, we completed the Nicaragua project and began to spread the wheelchair design and its technology to disabled people and their organizations in the Caribbean and Central and South America.

EVOLUTION OF THE DESIGN

The first prototype design for a Third World-appropriate wheelchair was based on features that wheelchair riders in the Western world often have learned to specify as modifications to the standard lightweight folding wheelchair to enable it to be used over rough terrain. When wheelchairs are used to climb curbs or follow rocky trails, for example, they bend and break if they are not properly reinforced. When they are propelled over rough ground, they lose traction and become impossible to push if they do not have pneumatic tires. Moreover, if they are any wider than necessary, they will not fit through many doorways; if they are too heavy, they will be hard to push and lift; if they do not fold, they will not fit in the aisle of a bus.

With rare exceptions, full-time users needing a single vehicle for both indoor and outdoor use have found nothing better than four-wheeled, rear-drive wheelchairs with the following features:

- *Width:* 24 inches maximum for a 16-inch or greater seat width.
- *Length:* 42 inches.
- *Weight:* 45 pounds for a fully equipped chair with armrest/fenders, brakes, footrests, handrims. Lightweight aluminum folding chairs, weighing as little as 30 pounds fully equipped, are now available at high cost.
- *Traction and Maneuverability:* A skilled rider of a four-wheeled, rear-drive chair can easily shift all of his or her weight to the drive wheels, giving full traction over rough terrain. When combined with pneumatic tires and a flexible frame, the four-wheeled, rear-drive chair gives excellent propellability and better stability than a three-wheeled chair of comparable width.
- *Ease of Assistance:* The rear-wheel drive chair can be tipped back on the rear wheels by an assistant and pushed or pulled over curbs and rough terrain.
- *Folds:* To a width of 12 inches or less. Easy disassembly of the chair by the rider has also been demanded by some users.
- *Accessibility:* The chair must not interfere with pulling close to a worktable or, for users who cannot stand, making lateral transfers into and out of the chair.
- *Durability:* The chair must stand up to the shock of ramming curbs and chuckholes and withstand rough treatment in all types of

transit. It must not be prone to breakdowns, which can strand the rider far from service facilities, and must perform with a minimum of routine maintenance. Commercial chairs vary widely in this regard.

These criteria—important for active wheelchair riders in the Western world—are particularly important for riders in Third World countries where doors are narrower, turning spaces are smaller, roads are rougher, curbs and steps are higher and less uniform, assistance in getting over obstacles is needed more often, wheelchairs must be lifted more often, and access to repairs is far more restricted.

Thus, my goal has been to design a wheelchair for manufacture and use in developing countries. It was to be at least as good as the best Western model but less expensive, made out of locally available materials, and built in workshops set up with a minimum of capital.

During the first year, I did most of the work on designing and revising prototypes for a Third World-appropriate wheelchair. After that, one of the disabled Nicaraguans, Omar Talavera, made significant contributions to the design. A visit in 1981 to Tahanan Walang Hagdanan (house with no stairs) in the Philippines, where 20 wheelchair riders had built more than 1,000 low-cost chairs, led to more significant changes in our design.

The major problems in developing a workable prototype stemmed from lack of materials and poor understanding of wheelchair use in Nicaragua. The economic situation in Nicaragua made it difficult, and sometimes impossible, for the wheelchair shop to purchase custom-made wheelchair parts from outside the country. We were forced to find ways to make wheelchair components out of standard Nicaraguan hardware, and the unavailability of materials in Nicaragua quickly began to dictate the design of our wheelchair. I had already decided to use zinc-plated electrical conduit instead of inch-sized seamed metal tubing, because the standard sizes of electrical conduit were more available in Nicaragua. The prototype design changed as I discovered what else was not available: hardened bolts, concentric tubing sizes, suitable ready-made hubs, and more. We are still trying to figure out how to make a high-resiliency, low-cost front wheel, but everything else is now made out of locally available materials.

My naivete about the life-style of disabled Nicaraguans caused one major change in the prototype. My original design called for a wooden folding seat, which allowed me to use a simpler and stronger folding mechanism than that in the average U.S. chair. That design had to be scrapped, however, because I had not taken into consideration the fact that, unlike wheelchair riders in the United States, most Nicaraguan wheelchair riders do not sit on cushions. A wooden seat would cause decubitus ulcers for people with spinal cord injuries. During the first year, I bought some cushions and tried to convince the group to use them. As the cushions wore out and needed replacement, I finally realized why most Nicaraguans would never use cushions—they cannot afford new ones.

I had also overlooked the need in Nicaragua for a folding wheelchair that allows the rider to fold the chair partially without getting out of it. The Nicaraguans partially fold their chairs to squeeze through the narrow doorways that are common in that country. We now have enough barrier-free buildings in the United States that this is not considered an essential feature.

As a result of these economic and practical problems, the current wheelchair design is almost completely original and is closely attuned to the needs of disabled people who live in rural areas and cannot afford anything but the cheapest wheelchairs.

THE FUTURE

The ability of the independent living center in Managua to proceed beyond prototype development into marketing of wheelchairs has been hampered by the problems the country has had in maintaining a general inventory of basic materials. Another problem is that the disabled people who run the independent living center and who grew up in poverty are not used to the concept of purchasing in bulk. Instead, they are used to buying today what they need today—as a result, they sometimes lose opportunities to buy needed materials when they are available.

The potential market for wheelchairs in Managua is great if measured by need. However, not many disabled Nicaraguans can afford to buy their own wheelchairs, even though the Managua-made wheelchair is much less costly than imported chairs. At present, materials for one wheelchair cost about U.S.$80, and 4–5 person-days are needed to complete each chair. The sales price is about U.S.$170. So far, 50 wheelchairs have been sold to private individuals in Nicaragua. Durability and ruggedness have been major characteristics built into our wheelchair's design, and it is hoped that the wheelchairs can be maintained indefinitely.

We have begun to spread what we have learned. Under the sponsorship of Appropriate Technology International, we held workshops in Jamaica, Peru, Costa Rica, Honduras, and California. Each mechanic completed a wheelchair and took it home to use as a model for production. A 150-page production manual, *Independence Through Mobility,* is now available from Appropriate Technology International. A new project, Appropriate Technology for Independent Living, has begun in California to carry on the development and dissemination of our wheelchair design worldwide.

Technological Innovation and Medical Devices

EDWARD B. ROBERTS

About 5 years ago, Robert Levy—then the director of the National Heart, Lung, and Blood Institute—and I cochaired a meeting that attempted to assess the state of knowledge about the development, dissemination, use, and acceptance of biomedical innovation. Having recently reread the proceedings of that meeting (Roberts et al., 1981), I perceive that much progress has been made during the past 5 years in our understanding of these critical aspects of medical technology.

I will illuminate the process of technological innovation in the field of medical devices by posing five questions. I would prefer to provide empirical answers to these questions and to use evidence drawn entirely from experiences with medical devices to identify what matters, what works and what does not work, and what the obstacles are to achieving more effective innovation. But the field of medical devices has not been researched as carefully or as thoroughly as one would have liked. Thus, I am going to draw upon some studies that have been done on innovations outside of the medical device field, on the few works that recently have been carried out on technological innovation in the medical device field, and on my 20 years of experience in this area.

WHAT IS TECHNOLOGICAL INNOVATION IN MEDICAL DEVICES?

Innovation can be classified in several ways, many of which are relevant to innovation of medical devices. For example, innovations in products, manufacturing processes, and modes of practice are all important. Both invention of new devices and modification of existing devices occur. Radical innovations that introduce dramatic new capabilities are important, as are incremental innovations in existing products and processes. Invention that is wholly original certainly takes place, but innovation also includes modifying, upgrading, and improving existing devices. Innovation also means adoption—taking a device that someone has developed previously and applying it to a different situation. A final way to distinguish among innovations is to recognize that some are based upon the application of new knowledge from scientific research, whereas others are clear cases of engineering problem solving, in which existing knowledge or techniques are applied to newly defined problems.

An overriding issue with these typologies is that our thinking about innovations in the medical field is dominated by images that come largely from the pharmaceutical industry. If most of us were asked to describe technological innovation in medical devices, we would speak about basic research that is carried out in large organizations and that generates fundamental knowledge used to create radical innovations in medical devices. Often, our managerial and policy approaches also reflect such images.

Yet, my personal experience, supported by the few relevant studies on innovation, indicates that the medical device field contradicts all of these images. Instead, innovation in medical devices is usually based on engineering problem solving by individuals or small firms, is often incremental rather than radical, seldom depends on the results of long-term research in the basic sciences, and generally does not reflect the recent generation of fundamental new knowledge. It is a very different endeavor from drug innovation, indeed.

Table 1 displays data gathered a number of years ago on innovations in 77 companies and in five different (all nonmedical) fields of activity (Myers and Marquis, 1969). In attempting to look at the amount of

TABLE 1   Technological Change Embodied in Successful Innovations

| | Percent Distribution[a] | | |
Degree of Inventiveness	Stage 1	Stage 2	Stage 3
Little	14	19	33
Considerable	41	50	48
Invention required	45	31	19

[a]$\chi^2 = 19.1; p < .001$.
SOURCE: Original data from Myers and Marquis (1969). Analysis from Utterback and Abernathy (1975).

TABLE 2   Degree of Functional Advance Embodied in British
Medical Equipment Innovations

Advance	Number	Example
First time provided to equipment user	10	Neonatal oxygen monitoring system
Major improvement in functionality	8	Radio pill telemetry system
Minor improvement	10	Miniaturization of radiography equipment
Failure	6	Nasal airways resistance tester
Total	34	

SOURCE: Shaw (1986).

technological change embodied in these innovations (degree of inventiveness), James M. Utterback of the Massachusetts Institute of Technology (MIT) and the late William J. Abernathy of the Harvard Business School clustered the data into three stages in the evolution of technology (Utterback and Abernathy, 1975). Stage 1 was emerging new technology; stage 2 was technology that was growing in adoption and use; and stage 3 was mature technology that was widely diffused and used. Utterback and Abernathy found that the characteristics of technological innovation depended upon the stage of evolution of the technology.

As depicted in Table 1, situations requiring original invention dominated stage 1 innovations only; much less invention typified innovations arising in stages 2 and 3. This suggests that an important dimension is whether the underlying technology of a particular medical device is newly emerging or not. If it is, then one should expect that a high degree of technological change will be required—possibly true invention and perhaps providing a real opportunity for basic scientific and engineering research to play an important role. If, however, a medical device is based on a technology that is well founded and widely diffused, the device innovation will likely merely involve upgrading, enhancing, and expanding current applications.

In a doctoral dissertation, Shaw (1986) shed light on this issue from the perspective of a small, randomly selected set of 34 innovations of medical equipment in Great Britain. The results of this study, summarized in Table 2, indicated that only 10 of the 34 innovations represented the first time that a particular function was provided to the equipment user (for example, a neonatal oxygen monitoring system). Of the remaining cases of (supposedly) significant innovations in medical devices, six were market failures (for example, a nasal airways resistance tester) and 18 were improvements on functions that had been previously available (8 were major improvements, such as the radio pill telemetry system; 10 were minor improvements, such as the miniaturization of radiography equipment). If Shaw's findings can be applied generally, then only a minority of medical device innovations bring a new functionality to health care providers.

In the same study, Shaw attempted to identify sources of key technological information that were embodied in the 34 innovations. Only 10 products were closely associated with original medical research. (Here, the term "associated" is used quite loosely, and includes all cases in which the innovation was developed in the course of carrying out medical research. Thus, the 10 cases were not necessarily devices that embodied recent results of original medical research.) For five innovations, clinical studies were an important source of ideas. But engineering and development were the major sources of innovative ideas for 19 products, clearly dominating the technological sources of ideas for medical device innovations.

WHO BRINGS ABOUT MEDICAL DEVICE INNOVATIONS?

It is commonplace in the field of innovation to talk about the importance of the relationship between the manufacturer and the user. The correct and well-supported presumption is that when a potential innovator focuses on needs and is attentive to the marketplace of prospective users, he or she can acquire insight into what products ought to be developed. As a consequence, resulting innovations are more likely to be successful.

One can go beyond this rather simplistic characterization, however. In many areas, including medical devices, the user is not merely a source of information about his or her needs to a manufacturer who innovates. Frequently, the user is the innovator. The innovative user not only defines a need, he or she also identifies the solution to that need. The innovative user often develops the initial innovation, places it into first clinical use, and makes copies or detailed specifications of the innovation available to other practitioners. Only later, in many cases, does a manufacturer acquire the user's innovation and begin to engage in the serious and important problems of commercial development—among them, engineering for manufacturing and for reliable field use, and service and volume scale-up.

Eric von Hippel of MIT has conducted a series of studies on sources of product innovations. His first four analyses focused on innovations in scientific instrumentation: gas chromatography, nuclear magnetic resonance, ultraviolet spectrophotometry, and transmission electron

TABLE 3   User Domination of Instrument Innovations

Category of Instruments	Percent User-Dominated	No. of User-Dominated	No. of Manufacturer-Dominated
Gas chromatography	82	9	2
Nuclear magnetic resonance	79	11	3
Ultraviolet spectrophotometry	100	4	0
Transmission electron microscope	79	11	3

SOURCE: von Hippel (1976).

microscopy (von Hippel, 1976). Despite a strict definition of what constitutes domination of an innovation, von Hippel concluded that 80 to 100 percent of the key innovations in these four scientific instruments were dominated by the user (Table 3). To qualify as user dominated, von Hippel insisted that the user had to have identified the need, developed the technical solution, put the solution into practice, and made the solution available to others in the field—all before a manufacturer played any role in these activities.

With the von Hippel study as a background, we can return to Shaw's recently completed study of British medical innovations (Shaw, 1986). Results were similar to those observed in von Hippel's study. For half of the British medical innovations (18 of 34), a prototype was developed and produced by a user. In another third of the cases (11 of 34), the innovative idea was transferred directly from the user to the manufacturer at the user's initiative, to satisfy the user's needs.

For only 4 of 34 devices was the innovation developed by a manufacturer who had performed market research to determine the nature and magnitude of a potential need, and then had developed a product to satisfy that need. In one case, the manufacturer went forward without the benefit of market research to push a technology that the manufacturer believed was desirable. Perhaps only coincidentally, that device was 1 of only 6 cases of market failure among the 34 medical innovations studied by Shaw.

Additional information about user and manufacturer initiatives for the 34 British medical equipment innovations was gathered by Shaw but not published with his dissertation. Four users started their own companies to manufacture their innovative devices. One new company was established by a potential user who was in contact with the innovative user. In six cases, the inventor contacted existing companies and asked them to develop and manufacture the invention. In four cases, a user approached an existing company after he had identified—but before he had invented—the solution. In one case, a government agency took the initiative and selected a firm to develop the device. In seven cases, there was an existing long-term relationship between an active user and a company working in the same field of medicine. For only 15 percent of the devices (5 of 34) did a company take the initiative in approaching a user for assistance in product development. And in even fewer cases (4 of 34) was the project initiated and carried out within the firm, without benefit of user relationships.

Another study by von Hippel and Finkelstein (1978) showed that user innovation can be encouraged or discouraged by medical equipment manufacturers. They demonstrated that the design of Technicon's auto-analyzer permitted nearly all of its test procedures to be developed by users, whereas DuPont's clinical analyzer had a closed design that produced dependency on DuPont's internal research and development professionals for supportive innovations.

Although the specific results may be somewhat different in a more comprehensive analysis of U.S. medical device innovations, these data clearly identify the locus of innovation for medical devices. The process of medical device innovation is dominated primarily by individuals, usually in academic and clinical settings, who are involved in the development and use of new technology in their respective fields. The role of the device manufacturer tends to be supportive and secondary—not primary—for most innovative medical devices.

For companies that are trying to innovate in medical fields, it is critical that they relate closely to the clinical scene. I recently completed a study of all new medical companies formed in Massachusetts between the years 1970 and 1975 (Hauptman and Roberts, 1987; Roberts and Hauptman, 1986, 1987). The study focused on the companies' activities in developing and marketing new products. A major finding was that the degree of clinical contact between those companies and, particularly, teaching hospitals was strongly correlated with the degree of technological innovation embodied in the products that the companies developed. It is nearly impossible for a biomedical company to be successful if it does not retain close ties to a clinical environment.

And yet, courting academicians as potential sources of new ideas is not an easy pathway to innovation. To illustrate this point, I rely on studies I performed a number of years ago using MIT faculty members in three departments—physics, electrical engineering, and mechanical engineering. Table 4 depicts what faculty members did with ideas that, in their judgment, had the greatest commercial potential (Roberts and Peters, 1981). Only about one-third took any strong steps to transfer their ideas to commercial manufacturers. Similar studies by researchers in MIT's two largest research laboratories replicated these findings (Peters and Roberts, 1969).

TABLE 4 Academicians' Exploitation of Their Commercially Oriented Ideas

Degree of Commercial Exploitation	Academic Ideas	
	No.	Percent
None	32	47
Weak	10	15
Strong	26	38
Totals	68	100

SOURCE: Roberts and Peters (1981).

More recently, I repeated the study with 75 full-time physicians at two major medical centers in the Boston area—one directly linked to a major medical school and the other a Veterans Administration hospital. More than half of the physicians (44 of 75) claimed to have come up with ideas that, if developed, would be worthwhile. Yet, less than half of those who had ideas had attempted to transfer them to commercial manufacturers. Of the 44 physicians who had ideas, 19 engaged in discussions with outside companies; 9 of them even entered into what they regarded as negotiations: 4 developed patent applications, and 1 formed a new company to try to commercialize the technological innovation. Academics at universities or in clinical settings may have productive ideas, but they infrequently exploit those ideas.

An important secondary finding in these studies was the lack of statistical correlation between the perceived potential benefits or medical importance of the ideas and the degree to which they are pushed toward commercial development. Routine academic ideas with little anticipated impact were as likely to get transferred to commercial firms as were exceptional ideas with excellent commercial prospects. Transfer depended more on the situation and the individual who developed the idea than on the quality of the idea itself. This was true both for MIT faculty members and for clinical and academic physicians.

Results of these studies permit us to conclude that inventive users are the principal driving force behind most medical device innovations, either as developers and initial implementers or in close association with commercial developers. Unfortunately, the data also demonstrate that a large number (perhaps most) of the potentially valuable ideas from users lie dormant in academia, in large part because academicians do not know about commercial technology transfer. This situation needs to be carefully examined in light of the increasingly favorable relationships between universities and industry. Such ties may permit a larger fraction of academic ideas to move toward commercial development.

WHICH COMPANIES CONTRIBUTE TO MEDICAL DEVICE INNOVATIONS?

An earlier study of innovation in nonmedical fields may provide some insight into the characteristics of firms that innovate in the field of medical devices. The information contained in Table 5 indicates that as new technologies emerge (stage 1), a number of small firms (each selling less than $10 million worth of products) dominate corporate sources of innovations. However, larger companies (those selling more than $100 million worth of products) account for most of the innovations during growth and development stages (stages 2 and 3) of technologies.

There is general misunderstanding in the United States and abroad about the relative roles of different-sized firms in the innovation process. Much of the talk about small companies being more innovative than large ones should be replaced by more accurate statements about how small companies are likely to be innovative at very early stages in the development of new technologies and how large companies are likely to be primary sources of innovation at later stages in the development of new technologies. Large companies that are particularly innovative have a special competitive edge for dominating later stages in a technology's evolution.

A similar phenomenon is likely to be true for innovation in the area of medical devices. Here, too, important differences in the timing and

TABLE 5   Firm Size and Successful Innovation as a Function of Stage of Technology

Size of Firms (Sales $ $\times 10^6$)	Stage of Evolution of Technology			
	Stage 1		Stages 2 and 3	
	No.	Percent	No.	Percent
Unclassified[a]	12	23	8	32
<10	18	34	0 (?)	0
10–100	6	12	2	8
>100	16	31	15	60

NOTE: A total of 77 firms were studied ($\chi^2 = 11.2$; $p < .01$).

[a]Unclassified firms are private companies that refused to provide sales data; they are all assumed to be doing less than $10 million in sales.

SOURCE: Original data from Myers and Marquis (1969). Analysis from Utterback and Abernathy (1975).

TABLE 6   Technology Development Milestones in Diagnostic Ultrasound

Year	Milestone	Developer	Market Introduction
1963	Commercial 2-D scanning	U. of Colo.	Physionics
1969	Mech. real time	U. of Colo.	Magnaflux
1972	Electronically switched real time	Dutch medical researchers	Organon Teknika
1973	Stored gray scale	Rohe Scientific	Rohe Scientific
1975	Electronic focus	Diagnostic Electronics	Diagnostic Electronics
1976	Microprocess controls	Searle Ultrasound	Searle Ultrasound
1977	Digital scan converter	Searle Ultrasound	Searle Ultrasound
1983	Computed sonography	Acuson	Acuson

SOURCE: Friar (1986).

type of a firm's innovations will depend on the size of the firm. These distinctions are critical for health care policymakers, since about 50 percent of U.S. medical device manufacturers have fewer than 20 employees. In a doctoral dissertation recently completed by John Friar (1986), eight major developmental milestones in the field of diagnostic ultrasound were identified. Table 6 lists these milestones; all occurred between 1963 and 1983 and were derived from careful assessment by experts. In only two cases did a large company (Searle) initially develop a key technological change. The three other cases in which companies were identified as innovators are intriguing: Each of the companies— Rohe Scientific, Diagnostic Electronics, and Acuson—were founded approximately at the time of development of the milestone that they subsequently introduced to the market.

Even when we focus on market introduction rather than technical development, the small firm remains the innovator during the early stages of a new technology. Physionics was a new firm that licensed ultrasound technology developed by the University of Colorado. Magnaflux was also a new firm that licensed an important development by the University of Colorado. Organon Teknika, a major corporation, licensed a development that came from a university in the Netherlands. As described in the preceding paragraph, Rohe Scientific, Diagnostic Electronics, and Acuson were all new firms that introduced their own new technologies.

These limited data suggest that small, innovative firms and university or hospital employees trying to satisfy their own needs as clinical or diagnostic users are the primary contributors to milestone developments in the medical device field. Personal experience and related research in other countries (Teubal et al., 1976) also support this conclusion.

HOW DO FDA REGULATIONS AFFECT MEDICAL DEVICE INNOVATION?

The importance of small firms to innovation in medical devices highlights concerns about the differential impact of Food and Drug Administration (FDA) regulations on large and small firms. A recent study of innovations in x-ray technology (Birnbaum, 1984) showed that increased FDA regulations led to decreased innovation of x-ray devices, especially by small firms. A 1986 study of innovation in contact lenses by the Office of Technology Assessment also expressed concern that small firms would be disproportionately affected by FDA regulations, particularly in the emerging technologies of soft and gas-permeable contact lenses (U.S. Congress, Office of Technology Assessment, 1987).

All this, however, does not mean that the FDA acts irresponsibly in its regulatory capacity. My recent study of medically oriented firms in Massachusetts indicated that the risk associated with use of these firms' new medical products—assessed by an independent medical panel—was significantly positively correlated with the degree of innovation embodied in a technology or in its application (Hauptman and Roberts, 1987). The more new technology that was embedded in a product, the greater was the product's assessed risk. This relationship held true for the first, second, and third new products that these companies introduced to the market, as well as for all of a company's products, taken together. The degree of assessed medical risk was less for new products classified as medical supplies than for new medical devices and pharmaceuticals; this relationship confirms logical expectations.

It is somewhat comforting to the skeptics among us to observe that the impact of FDA regulation is significantly correlated with the independent assessment of risk from new products: The greater the perceived medical risk, the more FDA intervention affected the companies involved in developing and marketing the product.

I believe this is the right direction for FDA activity, but there is an important negative side effect. The introduction of the Medical Devices Amendment in 1976 dramatically decreased the rate of new product introduction by young biomedical firms in Massachusetts (Hauptman and Roberts, 1987), and, although lacking empirical evidence, I suspect this also was true for young medical firms throughout the United

States. This may explain the negative correlation that exists for poorly financed biomedical firms between the extent to which a young firm is technologically innovative and the economic success of the company. Only in the medical field have I observed this relationship; in all other studies since 1964 there was a direct positive relationship between the degree of technological advance and the success of the firm. In the medical field, if the company is not sufficiently financed to overcome direct and indirect regulatory costs (particularly delays in generating product revenues), then being technologically innovative may be a curse rather than a benefit. This is a serious problem that should be addressed by both policymakers and managers.

It may be possible to speed up FDA review processes for smaller firms that suffer because of the costs needed to sustain themselves until market approval is obtained. This could be achieved by (1) preferential attention to, but not different standards for, applications from small companies; (2) expansion of FDA review staff; and (3) greater flexibility in accepting experimental data, especially overseas clinical trials.

WHAT IS THE ROLE OF THE LARGER COMPANY IN MEDICAL DEVICE INNOVATION?

A comprehensive study of the ultrasound industry provides a basis for information about expensive new medical devices (Friar, 1986). Of the 11 largest companies in the ultrasound device field, 9 entered the field by acquiring an innovator that had developed and commercialized some ultrasound technology. In four cases, the large company gained additional competitive technologies by further acquisitions. The only Japanese company on the list, Toshiba, entered the ultrasound field on its own and did not acquire outside technology as a major element of advancing its market position, a situation that contradicts our usual stereotype of Japanese firms as technologically acquisitive. In addition, Hewlett Packard entered the field based on its own technology but acquired Ekoline to strengthen its technological position.

If the larger company's role in medical device innovation is to acquire other firms (and, thereby, technological innovations), perhaps we should focus our attention exclusively on the activities of smaller firms. But large companies clearly dominate the medical device industry in sales. Most companies in the ultrasound industry are quite small, with 67 percent of them projected to have less than $5 million in sales in 1986. Only 20 percent of the firms are projected to sell more than $10 million worth of ultrasound equipment. The four largest companies are estimated to have 53 percent of the total U.S. market. Large sales are therefore concentrated in large companies that are not the original sources of most device innovations and that have usually acquired their technological base through licensing another firm's innovation or by acquiring that firm.

My own entrepreneurial experience in areas ranging from clinical diagnostics to medical information systems reaffirms conclusions drawn from the ultrasound example: Young, small firms dominate the initial stages of major innovations, and large companies advance principally through later acquisition of innovating small firms.

Large and small firms in the medical device industry play different roles: The small firm is frequently the early-stage innovator and is most jeopardized by the regulatory process. The large firm can afford the expense of the regulatory process, but is less likely to be affected because it is less often a key innovator. The patterns described here suggest that we need to support potentially synergistic relationships between large and small companies in the medical device industry. Potential ties that need to be examined and, perhaps, fostered range from sponsored research to venture capital to acquisition and alliances, and have been increasing rapidly in biotechnology and medical device fields in recent years. A recent study of 34 British medical equipment manufacturers showed a significant amount of collaboration between users and manufacturers and between small and large firms. A total of 25 manufacturers were involved in joint prototype testing and product evaluation and marketing, 19 manufacturers were involved in joint prototype development and product marketing, and 13 manufacturers were involved in joint prototype specification and marketing.

I believe that the potential benefits to companies and to society of various alliances between large and small firms are particularly promising in the field of medical devices. The evidence cited demonstrates that the primary roles of firms differ greatly as a function of their size. Younger, smaller firms offer technological innovations and display the entrepreneurial drive and commitment needed to bring a new medical device to initial use and early marketing. Large companies offer different resources: money, manufacturing capability, well-organized channels of distribution and field service, knowledge and experience for dealing with regulatory issues, and the opportunity to integrate multiple areas of technology. Large companies also contribute the potential for well-organized incremental technological improvements during growth and maturation of new medical technologies.

Explicit policy attention may be justified to strengthen beneficial relationships between large and small medical device firms. Areas for review might include the following: (1) the extent and criteria for awarding funds from medical devices, such as the National Institutes of Health's Small Business Innovation Research program; (2) tax treatment of expenses incurred by firms in appropriate collaborative research and development endeavors; and (3) federal funding of innovation stages beyond research, such as product development and research on market applications. Programs such as these exist in several countries that are trying to foster competitive industrial innovation. Additionally, strengthening ties between universities and large and small companies may enhance the innovation of medical devices and, thereby, benefit society.

REFERENCES

Birnbaum, P. H. 1984. The choice of strategic alternatives under increasing regulation in high technology companies. Academy of Management Journal 27(3):489–510.

Friar, J. H. 1986. Technology Strategy: The Case of the Diagnostic Ultrasound Industry. Ph.D. dissertation. Sloan School of Management, Massachusetts Institute of Technology, Cambridge.

Hauptman, O., and E. B. Roberts. 1987. FDA regulation of product risk and its impact upon young biomedical firms. Journal of Product Innovation Management 4(2):138–148.

Myers, S., and D. G. Marquis. 1969. Successful Industrial Innovations. NSF 69–17. Washington, D.C.: National Science Foundation.

Peters, D., and E. B. Roberts. 1969. Unutilized ideas in university laboratories. Academy of Management Journal 12(2):179–191.

Roberts, E. B., and O. Hauptman. 1986. The process of technology transfer to the new biomedical and pharmaceutical firm. Research Policy 15(3):107–119.

Roberts, E. B., and O. Hauptman. 1987. The financing threshold effect on success and failure of biomedical and pharmaceutical start-ups. Management Science 33(3):381–394.

Roberts, E. B., and D. Peters. 1981. Commercial innovation from university faculty. Research Policy 10(2):108–126.

Roberts, E. B., R. Levy, S. N. Finkelstein, J. Moskowitz, and E. I. Sondik, eds. 1981. Biomedical Innovation. Cambridge: MIT Press.

Shaw, B. F. 1986. The Role of the Interaction between the Manufacturer and the User in the Technological Innovation Process. Ph.D. dissertation. University of Sussex, Sussex, United Kingdom.

Teubal, M., N. Arnon, and M. Trachtenberg. 1976. Performance in innovation in the Israeli electronics industry: A case study of biomedical electronics instrumentation. Research Policy 5(4):354–379.

U.S. Congress, Office of Technology Assessment. 1987. Case Study No. 31: Contact Lenses. Washington, D.C.

Utterback, J. M., and W. J. Abernathy. 1975. A dynamic model of product and process innovation. Omega 3(6):639–656.

von Hippel, E. 1976. The dominant role of users in the scientific instrument innovation process. Research Policy 5(3):212–239.

von Hippel, E., and S. Finkelstein. 1978. Product designs which encourage or discourage related innovations by users: An analysis of innovation in automatic clinical chemistry analyzers. Working Paper. Sloan School of Management, Massachusetts Institute of Technology, Cambridge. (July).

Part 2
Current Trends

Federal Support of
Medical Device Innovation

LEO J. THOMAS, JR.

Every year, more than 80,000 Americans suffer permanently disabling but nonfatal injuries to the brain or spinal column. Many victims are young, just beginning their lives, and have much to offer society. It is estimated that direct and indirect costs of each of these disabling injuries is at least $100,000. The total cost to society adds up to an estimated $75 billion to $100 billion a year.

Reducing the costs of individuals disabled by injury is but one way that medical device innovation can benefit society. Development of new medical devices also offers hope to individuals suffering from arthritis, emphysema, heart disease, cancer, blindness, deafness, kidney malfunction, back pain, sleeping disorders, and a host of other health-related conditions.

Support for such innovation is in part a function of the partnership between private enterprise and the federal government, where each funds areas of research it is best qualified to support. Development of new medical devices depends on the broad base of biomedical knowledge—most of which is developed by public funds.

In 1986 the Commission on Engineering and Technical Systems of the National Research Council ordered a study to evaluate the state of engineering research in the United States. One of the seven areas studied was bioengineering.

In its final report (National Research Council, 1987, p. 88) the Bioengineering Research Panel highlighted eight areas in biomedicine that would benefit from further research. The areas are (1) systems physiology and modeling, (2) neural prostheses for human rehabilitation,

(3) biomechanics, (4) biomaterials, (5) biosensors, (6) metabolic imaging, (7) minimally invasive procedures, and (8) artificial organs. In several areas the application is already commercially attractive and some of the research support will come from private industry. In other areas, more basic knowledge needs to accumulate before commercial investment is likely. These areas would particularly benefit from public support of research.

SYSTEMS PHYSIOLOGY AND MODELING

Research in systems physiology and modeling derives from the modern engineer's need to describe complex systems by mathematical models. Such models can provide insight into the behavior of the system and can lead to experimentation that enhances our understanding of the system.

Living organisms are extremely complex systems. For example, a mature red blood cell performs some 2,000 biochemical reactions. And this is less complex than cells that are growing or dividing or cells that perform excretory or contracting functions. Integrating knowledge from cell biology, biochemistry, and physiology enables us to understand the living organism as a complex system and to predict the impact of man-made devices and remedies on the system.

Knowledge of physiology, particularly as expressed in models, has wide application in bioengineering. For example, Robert W. Mann has been conducting research on the human hip joint for several years. He has found that, although reported frictional coefficients in synovial joints are very low, a computer model of the human hip joint in simulated walking predicted a temperature rise within the joint of several degrees Celsius (Tepic et al., 1984). Dr. Mann confirmed this prediction with physical experiments on intact human hips dynamically loaded and articulated as in walking (Tepic et al., 1985), and demonstrated that heat shock proteins can be induced by the temperature increases predicted by the model (Madreperla et al., 1985).

Recently, Dr. Mann published the results of in vivo pressure measurements in the human hip joint (Hodge et al., 1986). A pressure-instrumented hip prosthesis monitored the pressure at 10 locations within the joint socket 253 times a second as the patient walked.

Results of such research help us understand initiation and progression of degenerative joint disease. This research has important implications for development of future prosthetic devices and for slowing or preventing the course of disease and thus for the several million people in the United States alone who suffer from degenerative hip disorders such as arthritis or avascular neurosis. Interestingly, support for Dr.

Mann's research did not come from the National Science Foundation (NSF) or the National Institutes of Health (NIH); it came mostly from the Department of Education.

NEURAL PROSTHESES FOR HUMAN REHABILITATION

The development of neural prostheses for human rehabilitation holds promise for victims of trauma, congenital defects, and acquired diseases such as cancer. More than 12 percent of Americans have some degree of physical disability, and each year more than 80,000 Americans sustain permanently disabling but nonfatal injuries to the brain or spinal column.

A new class of neural prostheses using integrated circuits is now in the early stages of development. Coupled with stable, biocompatible electrodes, these circuits can connect directly to the central and peripheral nervous systems. Inventions involving these devices, such as ear implants to bring sound to the neurologically deaf, offer great promise for improving the quality of life for some disabled individuals.

We are already seeing evidence that functional movement and bladder control can be restored to those who have suffered a stroke or spinal cord injury. In the future, we can anticipate development of devices that will give the blind a semblance of vision through electrical stimulation of the occipital center of the brain. We may even be able to restore functional movement and bladder control to those who have suffered a stroke or spinal cord injury.

BIOMECHANICS

Biomechanics deals with the response of living matter to physical forces. Such research has value in explaining and reducing both trauma—as occurs in accidents and sports—and long-term deterioration—which causes low back pain and osteoarthritis.

Biomechanics research can lead to the prevention of injuries. Injuries are the fourth leading cause of death in the United States and the leading cause of death for people age 1 through 44. In 1983 the National Center for Health Statistics estimated that there are 4.1 million preretirement years of life lost because of injuries in the United States per year. By contrast, 1.7 million years were lost to cancer and 2.1 million years to heart disease and stroke. However, only $112 million was spent for research on injury, whereas $998 million went to cancer research and $624 million to research on heart disease and stroke (National Research Council and Institute of Medicine, 1985).

Injury in America: A Continuing Public Health Problem, published in 1985 by the Institute of Medicine and the Committee on Trauma Research, Commission on Life Sciences, National Research Council (National Research Council and Institute of Medicine, 1985), suggests that the first step in understanding injury biomechanics is to understand how injuries occur. Yet, for most injuries this information is not available. Research is needed on the measurement of biomechanical responses, prevention of second injury to an injured area, determination of human tolerances to impact, and assessment of safety technology.

A thorough understanding of the neuromuscular control system will lead to improved artificial limbs and robotics, and perhaps to ambulatory systems for those disabled by injury. Biomechanics research, through an improved understanding of the interaction between blood flow and blood vessel walls, can help reduce the incidence of heart disease, atherosclerosis, and stroke—the leading causes of death in the United States.

Research on the biomechanics of the spinal column may help prevent certain types of back pain, studies of stresses in the lung can be used to treat emphysema victims, and biomechanics research on joints may help reduce arthritis joint degradation or assist in the development of permanent joint replacements.

BIOMATERIALS

Another priority for biomedical research is in the area of biomaterials. New opportunities to synthesize materials derive from the availability of polymers and macromolecules that, in addition to having specific engineering properties, can be designed to be compatible with the human body.

For example, biomedical engineers are conducting basic research on the interactions between biological molecules and cells in various environments. Because of the complexity of the interactions, however, much basic research is still needed.

BIOSENSORS

Biosensors are devices that convert biological information into an electronic signal that can be used for diagnosis or therapy. Research on biosensors leads to earlier disease detection and helps scientists better understand the body's natural sensors and actuators. Micromachining technology adapted from the microelectronics industry can lead to the development of smaller, more reliable, and more reproducible sensors. Chemical sensors suitable for use in laboratory and in vivo monitoring also require further research.

Research is necessary to make biosensors compatible with the human body and with signal processing systems. The goal is to produce minimally invasive sensors that permit diagnostic and therapeutic monitoring of a patient. The monitoring could be done at the patient's home and the information sent electronically to a hospital computer for review.

METABOLIC IMAGING

Metabolic imaging offers safe, powerful ways to see inside the body and includes such techniques as positron emission tomography (PET), magnetic resonance imaging (MRI), x-ray computed tomography, and ultrasound. In addition to physical information, biochemical information about natural substances and metabolites can now be obtained by some of these techniques. This field is highly dependent upon basic research on the physical and biochemical properties of body tissues and on integrative systems analysis.

MRI offers a good example of how federal funding for medical device innovation has affected the evolution of a technology and influenced the development of a medical device industry. In the early 1970s it was recognized that MRI could provide advantages over ionizing radiation by using radiowaves and powerful magnetic fields. It had the additional potential of providing excellent soft tissue contrast. These advantages would lead to the earlier detection of diseases and noninvasive, accurate pathologic diagnoses.

Balancing the potential advantages were some real barriers, including the high cost of magnetic resonance imagers and the difficult logistics of installation. MRI also required more physician time than alternative metabolic imagers, and its efficacy in clinical medicine compared to other imagers was unclear.

In this ambiguous situation, federal support of innovation in MRI was particularly important. For more than a decade, NIH supported research on MRI, biomedical application of MRI parameters, and biomedical application of magnetic resonance spectroscopy. For several years NIH had an active intramural program of research support for MRI applications. In addition, the National Cancer Institute funded programs to explore the use of MRI in studying the metabolism of normal and malignant cells and the effects of drugs on cell metabolism. The National Heart, Lung, and Blood Institute also funded several MRI-related extramural grants. In addition, the National Science Foundation supported a pioneering research effort on MRI at the University of California, Berkeley.

The effect of all this federal support over the decade of the 1970s was to provide a foundation that permitted industry to fund research on MRI applications. Today MRI is well accepted in the medical industry. Several manufacturers offer the machine for sale on a routine basis, ways are being found to cut the time required to produce an image, and costs are being managed so that MRI provides a good value for many situations.

MINIMALLY INVASIVE PROCEDURES

Minimally invasive procedures either replace or preclude the need for major surgery. For example, treatment for obstructed arteries usually involves open heart surgery and replacement of the obstructed arteries with segments of veins transplanted from other parts of the body.

A relatively new alternative to surgery is percutaneous transluminal coronary angioplasty. In this minimally invasive procedure, a catheter is threaded into the restricted vessel from an artery in the leg or arm and a small balloon at the end of the catheter is gently inflated to eliminate blockage without weakening or tearing the vessel.

Angioplasty is an excellent example of a new technology with social and economic benefits. It not only reduces discomfort and recovery time for patients but it is also less expensive. At present, approximately 250,000 cardiac bypasses are performed annually. At a cost of about $16,000 each, the total annual cost exceeds $4 billion (National Research Council, 1987, p. 95). Angioplasty costs about half that amount, and other minimally invasive procedures carry similar savings.

Angioplasty was developed with private funding by industry and is an example of the benefits that can accrue when private industry can justify the cost of research and development. In this case, there was a clear market for the catheters used in the procedure. That market amounted to $4 million in the early 1980s; in 1986 it had grown to $175 million, and is expected to reach $490 million in 1991.

It is important to keep in mind, however, that angioplasty would not have been developed if imaging techniques had not been available to permit the physician to see and maneuver the catheter. We therefore find that advances in one medical technology may lead to advances in others. Today, for example, the medical practitioner can perform percutaneous transluminal coronary angioplasty and other procedures such as lithotrypsy because relatively low-strength radiation can be used to see inside the human body.

ARTIFICIAL ORGANS

The final area of biomedical research emphasized by the Bioengineering Research Panel is artificial organs. Replacement of organs is in its infancy, and transplants and synthetic organs currently have limited effectiveness. The artificial heart program is exceedingly expensive, but other artificial organs—such as implanted insulin-producing cells for diabetics—may be less costly. In the future, multidisciplinary efforts combining biochemical and biomedical engineering should lead to synthetic systems capable of replacing natural, multifunctional organs in human beings.

As these new technologies develop, careful attention needs to be paid to the costs and benefits associated with introduction of new technologies and new medical devices. Such attention will encourage the effective and efficient use of new medical technologies and discourage costly and wasteful practices.

The enormous potential social benefit that would result from improving patient care and quality of life through research and development in these eight areas of bioengineering research is obvious. But there are also secondary social benefits—the potential of new technologies to improve the economic strength of the nation by creating jobs and having a favorable impact on the balance of trade.

Many of these new medical technologies may at first seem expensive, but productivity improvements can be foreseen. For example, a report of the Office of Technology Assessment (U.S. Congress, Office of Technology Assessment, 1984, p. 32) recalls that "in the mid-1950s and 1960s . . . a medical technologist could test a patient's blood for excess glucose manually, accomplishing six tests per hour. By 1983 one medical technologist, supervising the work of one machine, could turn out 1,800 individual tests per hour. But there was virtually no capital equipment in the mid-1950s instance, and about $400,000 in capital equipment in the 1983 case." And the process is continuing: Inexpensive devices have recently become available that permit diabetics to monitor their glucose levels at home, adjusting their therapy according to the results.

FEDERAL SUPPORT FOR BIOMEDICAL ENGINEERING RESEARCH

The effectiveness of steady, concentrated federal funding in developing medical technologies is illustrated by the roles of the National Institutes of Health, the Veterans Administration, and the Public Health Service in supporting the development of dialysis techniques for use in treating end-stage renal disease (ESRD), or kidney failure.

NIH funded early research on maintenance dialysis and on transplantation of kidneys. Annual funding for research on kidney and urinary tract disease at NIH increased from $47 million in 1976 to $90 million in 1982. These funds contributed significantly to the development of hollow-fiber dialyzers, the efficient enhancement of flat-plate dialyzers, the introduction of "single-needle" dialyzers, the determination of dietary protein levels for dialysis patients, the establishment of a national registry of patients on dialysis, the development of absorbents for uremic wastes, the development of a portable artificial kidney, the prevention and treatment of chronic bone pain and bone fractures in patients, the treatment of chronic anemia in patients, and the development of the concept of hemofiltration.

Other federal policies were also crucial to the development of dialysis technology. In the early 1970s, the federal government decided that dialysis would be reimbursed by government medical programs. With this assurance, and the foundation provided by publicly funded research, private funding of dialysis research increased and devices for this market were developed. Before that assurance, manufacturers had considered this an orphan device field—one with insufficient market potential to justify the private expense of developing products. Today, kidney dialysis is a thriving business.

At present, U.S. support for fundamental research in biomedical engineering is relatively small and scattered throughout the federal government. Because biomedical engineering is a multidisciplinary activity, it does not often conform to traditional boundaries of policy issues and research programs. Biomedical engineering, therefore, may lack the organizational focus that oncology, for example, finds in the National Cancer Institute.

Federal support for biomedical engineering research is spread across a number of agencies: the National Science Foundation, the National Institutes of Health, the National Bureau of Standards, the Departments of Energy (DOE) and Education, and the Veterans Administration, among others. In addition, support for biomedical engineering research frequently is spread among different units within agencies.

It is difficult to find reliable estimates for federal expenditures supporting biomedical engineering research. For example, the NSF Engineering Directorate funded programs in biochemical and biomass engineering research, biotechnology, and aid to the handicapped at a combined $9.4 million in fiscal year 1985. In addition, NSF provided funds for bioengineering research through its Industry-University Cooperative Research Project. NSF support for biochemical and biomedical engineering may have totaled $12 million in fiscal year

1985. The biomedical engineering portion of this $12 million, however, was relatively small.

An analysis of NIH, NSF, and DOE grants active in early 1983 indicated that funds totaling nearly $50 million supported research on diagnostic imaging. This support was scattered through various institutes and agencies and covered a wide variety of subjects.

The National Institutes of Health, the principal agency of the U.S. government for support of biomedical research, has an overall budget of $5.5 billion per year. This research investment provides a rich source of new scientific knowledge that creates opportunities for the development of new medical devices. However, investment in the fundamental areas of biomedical engineering constitutes only about 1 percent of the NIH budget. At NIH, few engineers are represented on groups that award extramural grants. NIH's Intramural Research Program funds $660 million of research by in-house investigators each year; only $11 million of this budget goes to the Biomedical Engineering and Instrumentation Branch. Less than 5 percent of the 5,000 people with advanced degrees who conduct research at NIH are bioengineers or are from a bioengineering-related discipline.

Because of increased competition for limited research resources, government agencies involved in biomedical engineering research have begun to shift from a philosophy in which research grants were seen as instruments for investment to one in which grants are considered a means to procure a product. Such research may not be best accomplished in government and university laboratories, and a promising alternative has been developed. In the early 1980s, the federal government established the Small Business Innovation Research (SBIR) program. In fiscal year 1983, NIH expended $7.3 million in the SBIR program. An analysis conducted by the Office of Technology Assessment showed that approximately 40 percent of NIH's Small Business Innovation Research awards supported medical device applications (U.S. Congress, Office of Technology Assessment, 1984, p. 86).

High-risk bioengineering research projects—fundamental research that may significantly benefit society but carries a large risk of failure— are important, but such projects are not often funded by federal agencies. One way to remedy this is for each agency to earmark funds for high-risk research. The NSF has already established such a program. Alternatively, awards can be given to investigators based on their research histories. Such awards may provide successful researchers with the opportunity to conduct high-risk research.

Federal funding of biomedical engineering research also supports education and training of young biomedical engineers. Over the past decade, biomedical engineering students have represented less than 2 percent of all engineering students in both master's and doctoral degree programs. During this time, there has been a decline in the number of doctoral students and an increase in the number of students enrolled in terminal master's degree programs in biomedical engineering. The decline of Ph.D. students may reflect a loss of students to medical schools or other fields that have better research funding. There is a clear need to train more young Ph.D.-level engineers who understand the major principles of biology, medicine, and other relevant scientific disciplines.

Advanced-degree engineering students may not be choosing biomedical engineering because career opportunities are unclear. As public and private support of research and development in biomedical engineering becomes stronger, career opportunities would become evident, bringing talented students into the field.

CONCLUSION

Numerous research opportunities exist in at least eight biomedical engineering fields, promising significant social and economic benefits. But private industry will do only part of the necessary work. Federal support for basic bioengineering research must continue to provide a knowledge base that medical device manufacturers can use to make decisions about developing and marketing new technologies.

Federal support for bioengineering research is scattered among agencies, insufficient to fund many worthwhile projects, and not well coordinated. A mechanism should be created to review and coordinate federal programs which support bioengineering research. The Bioengineering Research Panel recently recommended that coordination of research programs in biomedical engineering could be improved through creation of an interagency body that has the support of senior administrators in each participating agency (National Research Council, 1987, p. 109).

It may also be worthwhile for NIH to establish an interdisciplinary center for biomedical research that would be similar in concept to the NSF's Engineering Research Centers. The Bioengineering Research Panel also recommended that individuals who rank grant proposals and award research funds in NIH and NSF consider funding projects that, although they have great potential for significant results, might also have a high risk of failure.

Finally, the Bioengineering Research Panel suggested that there be a permanent advisory body to assess biomedical engineering research opportunities and needs, review relevant agency projects, and identify new and changing program needs.

In closing, I would like to remind readers not to lose sight of the great commercial potential in biomedical engineering. The overall U.S. market for biomedical engineering devices and systems in 1987 is estimated to be over $20 billion, and parts of that market are growing at annual rates ranging from 10 to 25 percent. New opportunities in the eight areas of biomedical engineering could add considerably to that market.

For the sake of basic research that could alleviate human suffering and reduce the costs of medical care, and for the potentially large commercial markets for products resulting from such research, I hope to see increased cooperation among federal agencies funding basic bioengineering research and between those agencies and the medical devices industry.

REFERENCES

Hodge, W. A., R. S. Fijan, K. L. Carlson, R. G. Burgess, W. H. Harris, and R. W. Mann. 1986. Contact pressures in the human hip joint measured *in vivo*. Proceedings of the National Academy of Sciences USA 83(May):2879–2883.

Madreperla, S. A., B. Louwerenburg, R. W. Mann, C. A. Towle, H. J. Mankin, and B. V. Treadwell. 1985. Induction of heat-shock protein synthesis in chondrocytes at physiological temperatures. Journal of Orthopaedic Research 3:30–35.

National Research Council. 1987. Directions in Engineering Research: An Assessment of Opportunities and Needs. Engineering Research Board. Washington, D.C.: National Academy Press.

National Research Council and Institute of Medicine. 1985. Injury in America: A Continuing Public Health Problem. Committee on Trauma Research, Commission on Life Sciences. Washington, D.C.: National Academy Press.

Tepic, S., T. Macirowski, and R. W. Mann. 1984. Simulation of mechanical factors in human hip articular cartilage during walking. Pp. 834–839 in Summer Computer Simulation Conference, Boston, Mass., July 26–27, 1984. La Jolla, Calif.: Society for Computer Simulation.

Tepic, S., T. Macirowski, and R. W. Mann. 1985. Experimental temperature rise in human hip joint in vitro in simulated walking. Journal of Orthopaedic Research 3:516–520.

U.S. Congress, Office of Technology Assessment. 1984. Federal Policies and the Medical Device Industry OTA-H–229 (October). Washington, D.C.

Private Investment in Medical Device Innovation

ANTHONY A. ROMEO

Medical device innovations have been developed by a mix of private and public funding. Of course, support from the private sector has been motivated, at least in part, by a quest for profits. This prospect has spurred the research and development (R&D) and risk-taking necessary for innovation.

This paper examines some of the business considerations that lie behind private investment in medical device innovation. To date, business investment decisions have reflected an optimism about the rich technological opportunities for developing new products and the attractive sales potential in an apparently expanding market. But are changes in the economic, legal, or regulatory environment likely to destroy the incentives for business investment? Is federal support of private investment called for?

DECISIONS ABOUT R&D

R&D is an investment. Decisions about R&D funding can be approached, in principle, like other investment decisions. One compares costs and returns and invests in a project, or set of projects, if the expected returns are deemed satisfactory. Such an evaluation is particularly difficult for R&D. In essence, investment in R&D is an investment in knowledge (Arrow, 1962). Outcomes cannot be readily specified in advance. Such decisions require the commitment of existing real resources to an uncertain future.

Creative people have developed a variety of techniques for making such decisions. All involve balancing market and technological criteria, and each technique balances the criteria and adjusts for uncertainty in various ways. Techniques range from formal models that rely primarily on quantitative methods to informal models that rely primarily on personal judgment. The R&D literature is full of discussion advocating one approach or another (Coopers and Lybrand, 1986; Kay, 1979). There is no clear consensus, but it appears that in practice most firms lean toward a more judgmental approach. There is much reliance on heuristics and rules-of-thumb.

This would especially seem to be the case in the medical devices industry. The industry has a high population of small firms, and small firms generally tend to eschew the more formal decision-making techniques. Moreover, in fast-changing industries such as this, much of the quantitative data available are obsolete or irrelevant. Intuition may be crucial.

Yet, in all cases, the evaluation will consider a variety of factors that determine the technical possibilities and market potential of the innovation. These factors will vary within segments of the medical devices industry. Moreover, interpretation of the evidence will vary among firms according to personal judgment and attitudes. But there are factors that are likely to be broadly relevant to all firms in the industry, and these are worth considering in detail.

TECHNICAL FACTORS

Technical factors determine the ease with which an innovation can be developed and brought to the market. There are two key technical factors that distinguish development efforts in the medical devices industry. One is the nature of the scientific base on which development builds. The other is the regulatory environment in which development occurs.

Investments in R&D build on an existing scientific base. That base seems to hold considerable promise for this industry. For example, potential applications in biotechnology are generating considerable excitement, and technological advances in materials and microelectronics seem likely to find further applications. As any venture capitalist will tell you, there is no shortage of ideas for new medical devices.

Strengthening the base will expand technological horizons and opportunities, effectively reducing the cost of achieving specific performance objectives. The future strength of the scientific base in turn depends heavily on the federal government, which is by far the major source of funds for basic scientific research. Private industry cannot be relied on to do much basic research; the payoff from such activity is too distant and elusive to be justifiable in a business environment that is committed to short-term results. Only larger firms or speculators will make such commitments. Even then, the amounts spent on basic research will be small relative to applications-oriented R&D.

Federal investment in basic research, then, is clearly a complement and a spur to private R&D efforts (Nelson, 1976). In the case of applied research, however, federal funds are occasionally seen as a substitute for private funds. As such, they are often viewed as an inefficient use of scarce resources. But there is little convincing evidence on this score. Indeed, a recent study suggests that federally funded industrial R&D has actually tended to stimulate private spending (Levy and Terleckyj, 1985). Again, the principle is the same; such research provides a base on which further efforts can build.

Certainly, the research base in universities, however funded, has contributed to innovation in medical devices. Examples abound of cases in which university research was the starting point for a new device. For example, Technicon's continuous-flow Auto Analyzer, which was introduced 30 years ago, had its origins in the work of a researcher at Case Western Reserve University (E. Whitehead, Development of Technicon's Auto Analyzer in the paper "Inventing Medical Devices: Five Inventors' Stories," this volume). Today, many businesses try to tap the base of knowledge and expertise in universities. Although it is difficult to judge the overall economic effects, there is no doubt that universities and businesses are often tied together in the innovation process. As an illustration of this trend, consider the glucose sensor now marketed by Baxter Travenol. This sensor was invented by a research team at Oxford University, developed into a prototype model at Cranfield Institute of Technology, and then brought to commercial quality by Genetics International, Inc., which had funded the academic work.

Any stimulative effects of a strong research base will be influenced by the ease with which the base is tapped. Certain institutional features could affect private efforts to use the base. For example, if the information is widely dispersed or difficult to gain access to, then opportunities may be missed. More directly, the producers of new knowledge may decide to raise its price. For example, universities now seem to be becoming more marketwise, guarding expertise and patents more carefully than they have in the past. Some are forming companies to exploit their research discoveries.

Even with a strong scientific base, innovation will require corporate in-house efforts to develop a device and bring it to market. For medical devices, these efforts are complicated by regulatory requirements.

Most notable are the 1976 Medical Devices Amendments to the Food, Drug and Cosmetics Act.

The possible effects of the 1976 Medical Devices Amendments have been discussed extensively (U.S. Congress, Office of Technology Assessment, 1984). Of course, because the actual regulatory procedures have been in effect for a relatively short time, there is little hard evidence about their effects on innovation. What evidence exists is anecdotal or is based on parallels drawn with the 1962 Drug Amendments to the Food, Drug and Cosmetics Act, whose effects also have been extensively, if not conclusively, investigated (Grabowski, 1976, 1983; Grabowski et al., 1978; Peltzman, 1974; Schwartzman, 1950; Wardell and Lasagna, 1975).

The principles involved, however, are clear. Certainly, if a device is placed in class III and requires "premarket approval," the costs of innovation are likely to be higher than for devices placed in classes I and II. These are costs of both time and physical resources. The prospects of having to incur these costs will tend to discourage corporate investment in class III device innovation (Harris and Associates, 1982; Arthur D. Little, Inc., 1982; U.S. Congress, Office of Technology Assessment, 1984).

Increased uncertainty may be even more critical than actual costs. To the extent that regulation increases uncertainty, it will discourage activity among the many managers who are, by their nature, averse to risk. Of course, as manufacturers gain experience with the regulatory process and confidence in their ability to deal with it, uncertainty is reduced and its discouraging effects lessened. However, this will require consistency and stability in the regulatory process. Constant changes in rules and interpretations can be quite discouraging.

Regulatory concerns can also affect the direction of activity. For example, there could be a bias toward categories of devices that do not require an involved approval process. This could result in a preference for developing diagnostic instead of therapeutic devices. Or it could lead to a strategy of small, incremental changes resulting in the production of devices that can be classified as "substantially equivalent" to devices in use before 1976. Smaller and shorter-term projects will also be preferred because of a desire to avoid the uncertainty inherent in long-term projects.

Regulatory pressure may indirectly affect innovation by altering the internal structure of the medical devices industry. At present, most firms in the industry are small, but larger firms may be able to cope more effectively with regulation (Harris and Associates, 1982; Arthur D. Little, Inc., 1982; Schifrin with Rich, 1984). Large firms can better afford the costs of regulation and seem to learn more quickly how to manage the regulatory process. They are secure enough financially to weather some failures and are better able to appropriate the benefits of success. Even in the absence of regulation, the natural evolution of "high-tech" industries may result in fewer and larger medical device manufacturers.

A change in structure of the industry may change the nature of innovation. Many would argue that it is smaller firms that produce most of the significant innovations (Edwards and Gordon, 1984; Gellman Research Associates, 1982). Certainly, smaller firms possess more entrepreneurial spirit. Although there are many articles in the business literature explaining how large firms can maintain entrepreneurial flair (for example, how they can practice "intrapreneurship" [Pinchot, 1985]), the environment for innovation in most large firms will be different than that in small ones.

In large firms, the process of innovation will be brought under the control of general management. Technological products will be more closely tuned to perceived market needs and wants. There will be less of a tendency to try to create new markets or complete new products and more of an emphasis on refining and improving current products (Ansoff, 1987; Porter, 1980). Such a pattern is evident, for example, in the now well-established wheelchair market (Shepard and Karon, 1984).

Note, however, that this process does not necessarily result in more or less innovation, just a different form of it.

MARKET FACTORS

Ultimately, the innovator's success will be determined by the market's reaction to the innovation. Will customers buy a new device in the quantities and at a price sufficient to generate a profit? To justify investing in innovation, the answer should be yes. But I suspect that, for many innovators, the answer has been based more on faith than on analysis. The industry has been more technology-driven than market-driven. The attitude often seems to have been that a particular technical idea is so good that there has to be a market out there for it.

Certainly, the market for medical devices looks attractive. If one hired some of the major business consulting firms to gauge market attractiveness using portfolio models, the industry would probably score highly (Porter, 1985). Growth prospects look good, demographic trends seem favorable, and demand for the underlying product—health—will remain strong. In this context it is easy to understand the enthusiasm of scientists-entrepreneurs, of venture capitalists, and of large, established firms seeking to diversify from low-growth markets into health care. But this enthusiasm should be tempered with an awareness of several additional factors.

First, the attractions of the health care market are widely known. As firms rush to take advantage of obvious opportunities, markets or market segments will become crowded. Large firms seeking to expand into new market segments, entrepreneurs with a good idea, and foreign firms eyeing the vast U.S. health care market will all be there. All this interest may be good for the consumer, but the manufacturer may find a crowded market a difficult one in which to make profits. For example, this seems to be the case in certain areas of biotechnology (Imman, 1987).

Second, developing a new product that embodies some technological advance will not be enough. The firm that develops the product may not be able to capture its full benefits, and imitators may gain some of the profits. Additionally, there may be alternative products with a legitimate claim to performing the same function. Convincing consumers of the superiority of a new product may prove difficult and costly. And, in a fast-moving environment, such superiority can dissipate quickly. Marketing skills will be crucial, and small firms may find they lack the expertise to compete on this basis.

Liability laws will also affect medical device manufacturers' decisions. Many will be reluctant to introduce innovations which present substantive liability risks. Also, the regulatory system will have some effects on market attractiveness. A number of studies have been done on the effects of Certificate of Need and Prospective Payment System regulations on the diffusion of innovations (Cromwell and Kanak, 1982; Hillman and Schwartz, 1985; Russell, 1979; Sloan et al., 1986; Wagner et al., 1982). They suggest that, in some situations, regulation may have discouraged the adoption of high-cost and quality-enhancing innovations. If market potential is limited in this way, expected returns are reduced and private investment in innovation is likely to be discouraged.

But some studies have suggested that the Prospective Payment System may stimulate the adoption of cost-saving innovation (Anthony, 1985; Romeo et al., 1984; Sloan and Valvona, 1986). The effect could be complicated (Garrison and Wilensky, 1986), but there could be redirection of some investments from new technologies that are quality-enhancing to those that are predominantly cost-saving. This seems to have been the case for hollow-fiber dialyzers, for example (Rettig, 1980).

Changes in reimbursement can affect the direction of investment in other ways, too. For example, some recent reimbursement changes are interpreted as creating pressures on hospitals and physicians to shift the locus of care from hospitals to the home. To the extent that health care treatment modalities and equipment are location-specific, their ability to attract investment will change accordingly. In the case of kidney dialysis, reimbursement changes have supported continuous ambulatory peritoneal dialysis, a home-based procedure, and have led to increased research and development on devices associated with that form of treatment (Romeo, 1984).

Again, the specter of uncertainty arises. Firms can adjust to changes in reimbursement procedures, changes in legal interpretations, and changes in the mix of health care needs. They will respond by choosing a portfolio of investments that are tuned to the market environment. But what firms deal with less effectively is uncertainty. Not knowing what will happen or not understanding leads to a reluctance to invest.

CONCLUSIONS

Given the many factors affecting innovation, can we be assured that there is enough, or the right kind, of innovation in medical devices today? Is increased federal support for medical device research and development necessary or appropriate?

Discussion of innovation of medical devices has largely focused on the negative incentives for innovation created by government regulation. Certainly, there is reason to believe that some regulatory activities may diminish investment in innovation. From this conclusion, many go on to argue that regulatory disincentives ought to be compensated for: R&D in the industry should be subsidized. There are a variety of ways to generate R&D incentives and a variety of ways to lessen the negative effects of reimbursement policies. But to advocate these, one must be confident of the basic premise that too little is being invested now in innovation.

Let us examine that premise. Economists often argue that private firms tend, from a social perspective, to underinvest in R&D (Arrow, 1962). From society's point of view, firms should invest in R&D as long as the social benefits—i.e., the benefits to society at large—exceed the costs. However, the private firm will invest in R&D only as long as its private benefits exceed costs.

These two criteria diverge when private and social benefits diverge, and there is ample evidence that they do (Mansfield et al., 1977; Robert R. Nathan Associates, 1978; Tewksbury et al., 1980). Innovators rarely appropriate the full benefits of their innovation. Benefits are sometimes passed on to consumers and suppliers and may be secured by imitating competitors. Thus, there are circumstances when an investment in R&D would yield an attractive social return but an inadequate private return. In such cases, the private firm does not invest, even though the investment would be valuable to society.

This situation seems to merit government intervention to encourage research and development. This reasoning lies behind several government programs, including the recent federal tax credit for incremental research and development (Eisner et al., 1984).

But this argument relies on defining benefits to consumers and to society on the basis of their willingness to pay for a good or service (Eisner et al., 1984; Mansfield, 1986), which is determined by reference to market prices. When market prices reflect value to consumers, this argument makes good sense. In the health care field, however, it is unclear that prices are a reasonable reflection of consumer value. Market valuations—and the corresponding signals for investment in R&D—are greatly affected by insurance provisions, consumer ignorance, physician preferences, and other factors. Relying on consumers' willingness to pay may be misleading. Indeed, one could argue that the alleged overspending on medical care that has prompted many of the recent changes in reimbursement policies may have created an excessively strong signal to invest in R&D. New incentives may be simply countering previous inappropriate signals.

Overall, the basis for arguing for industry-wide federal subsidies in support of medical device research and development is rather weak. With R&D spending in the industry at twice the national average and with the industry continuing to show vigorous growth, justification of federal subsidies would require more proof than the argument that regulation creates disincentives (Geiser, 1986; Mannen and Campbell, 1985; Pollard et al., 1986). We need careful study and clear evidence on innovation activities in the medical device industry.

But what about the direction of medical device research and development? Even if the overall magnitude is high, will socially appropriate sorts of innovation be done?

Clearly, private investment will tend to be directed toward making profits, and private firms will respond to market signals. Where these are weak, little investment will flow. There are, therefore, likely to be "orphan" devices and, more generally, imbalances in innovation. To some extent, government also sends signals to manufacturers. For example, the decision to fund the end-stage renal disease program stimulated considerable research in dialysis equipment (Romeo, 1984). But, as suggested earlier, there is no assurance that market or government signals in health care accurately reflect social values or that they will stimulate a balanced mix of investments. Presuming that a definition of social appropriateness can be agreed upon, government intervention may be required to achieve the desired balance. However, we need much more study before we can determine the precise ways in which such a balance can best be accomplished.

REFERENCES

Ansoff, H. I. 1987. Strategic management of technology. Journal of Business Strategy 7(3):28–39.

Anthony, F. H. 1985. New product opportunities with DRGS. Hospital Pharmacy 20(10):10–11.

Arrow, K. 1962. Economic welfare and the allocation of resources for inventions. Pp. 609–624 in The Rate and Direction of Inventive Activity. National Bureau of Economic Research. Princeton, N.J.: Princeton University Press.

Coopers and Lybrand. 1986. Evaluating R and D and New Product Development Ventures: An Overview of Assessment Methods. Report to the U.S. Department of Commerce, Office of Productivity, Technology and Innovation, Washington, D.C.

Cromwell, J., and J. Kanak. 1982. The effects of prospective reimbursement programme on hospital adoption and service sharing. Health Care Financing Review 4(2):67.

Edwards, K. L., and T. J. Gordon. 1984. Characterization of innovations introduced on the U.S. market in 1982. Report to the Office of Advocacy, U.S. Small Business Administration, Washington, D.C.

Eisner, R., S. Albert, and M. Sullivan. 1984. The new incremental tax credit for R&D. National Tax Journal 37(June):1971–1983.

Garrison, L. P., and G. R. Wilensky. 1986. Cost containment and incentives for technology. Health Affairs 5(2):46–58.

Geiser, N. S. 1986. The evolving medical device industry: 1976 to 1984. Medical Device and Diagnostic Industry (November):51–54.

Gellman Research Associates. 1982. The Relationship Between Industrial Concentration, Firm Size and Technological Innovation. Report prepared for the U.S. Small Business Administration. Washington, D.C.: Gellman Research Associates.

Grabowski, H. G. 1976. Drug Regulation and Innovation. Washington, D.C.: American Enterprise Institute.

Grabowski, H. G. 1983. Studies on Drug Substitution, Patent Policy and Innovation in the Pharmaceutical Industry. Report prepared for the National Science Foundation.

Grabowski, H. G., J. M. Vernon, and L. C. Thomas. 1978. Estimating the effects of regulation on innovation: An international comparative analysis of the pharmaceutical industry. Journal of Law and Economics 21:133–163.

Harris and Associates. 1982. A Survey of Medical Device Manufacturers. Report to the Food and Drug Administration, Bureau of Medical Devices. Washington, D.C.: Harris and Associates.

Hillman, A. L., and J. S. Schwartz. 1985. The adoption and diffusion of CT and MRI in the United States: A comparative analysis. Medical Care 23(November):1283–1294.

Imman, B. 1987. Biotech's acquired income deficiency syndrome. Business (February):80–83.

Kay, N. M. 1979. Corporate decision-making for allocations to research and development. Research Policy 8:46–69.

Levy, D. M., and N. E. Terleckyj. 1985. Trends in Industrial R&D Activities in the

United States, Europe and Japan, 1963–1983. Report to the National Science Foundation, Washington, D.C.

Arthur D. Little, Inc. 1982. Cost of Compliance with Good Manufacturing Practices Regulations by the Medical Devices Industry. Final report for the Food and Drug Administration, Department of Health and Human Services. Washington, D.C.: Arthur D. Little, Inc.

Mannen, T., and P. Campbell. 1985. Interim funding suggested for specific kinds of new technologies prior to DRG adjustments. Interview. Review. Federation of American Hospitals 18(4):44–47.

Mansfield, E. 1986. The R&D tax credit and other technology policy issues. American Economic Review 76(2):190–194.

Mansfield, E., J. Rapoport, A. Romeo, S. Wagner, and G. Beardsley. 1977. Social and private rates of return from industrial innovations. Quarterly Journal of Economics 91:221–240.

Robert R. Nathan Associates. 1978. Net Rates of Return on Innovations, vols. 1 and 2. Report to the National Science Foundation, Washington, D.C.: Robert R. Nathan Associates.

Nelson, R. R. 1976. Institutions supporting technical advance in industry. American Economic Review 76(2):186–189.

Peltzman, S. 1974. Regulation of Pharmaceutical Innovation: The 1962 Amendments. Washington, D.C.: American Enterprise Institute.

Pinchot, G. 1985. Intrapreneuring: Why You Don't Have to Leave the Corporation to Become an Entrepreneur. New York: Harper & Row.

Pollard, M. R., G. S. Persinger, and J. G. Perpich. 1986. Data watch: Technology innovation in health care. Health Affairs 5(2):135–147.

Porter, M. E. 1980. Competitive Strategy. New York: The Free Press.

Porter, M. E. 1985. Competitive Advantage. New York: The Free Press.

Rettig, R. A. 1980. The politics of health cost containment: End stage renal disease. Bulletin of the New York Academy of Medicine 56:115–138.

Romeo, A., J. Wagner, and R. Lee. 1984. Prospective reimbursement and the diffusion of new technologies in hospitals. Journal of Health Economics 3(1):1–24.

Romeo, A. A. 1984. The Hemodialysis Equipment and Disposables Industry (Health Technology Case Study 32). OTA-HCS-32. Washington, D.C.: U.S. Congress, Office of Technology Assessment.

Russell, L. 1979. Technology in Hospitals: Medical Advances and Their Diffusion. Washington, D.C.: Boorhinge Institute.

Schifrin, L. G., with W. J. Rich. 1984. The Contact Lens Industry: Structure, Competition, and Public Policy (Health Technology Case Study 31). OTA-HCS-31. Washington, D.C.: U.S. Congress, Office of Technology Assessment.

Schwartzman, D. 1950. Innovation in the Pharmaceutical Industry. Baltimore: John Hopkins University Press.

Shepard, D. S., and S. L. Karon. 1984. The Market for Wheelchairs: Innovations and Federal Policy (Health Technology Case Study 30). OTA-HCS-30. Washington, D.C.: U.S. Congress, Office of Technology Assessment. (This case study was performed as part of OTA's assessment of Federal Policies and the Medical Devices Industry.)

Sloan, F. A., and J. Valvona. 1986. Prospective payment for hospital capital by Medicare: Issues and options. Health Care Management Review 11(2):25–33.

Sloan, F. A., J. M. J. Perrin, and K. W. Adamache. 1986. Diffusion of surgical technology. Journal of Health Economics 5:31–61.

Tewksbury, J. G., M. S. Crandall, and W. E. Crane. 1980. Measuring the societal benefits of innovation. Science 209(August):658–662.

U.S. Congress, Office of Technology Assessment. 1984. Federal Policies and the Medical Devices Industry. OTA-H–230. Washington, D.C.: U.S. Congress, Office of Technology Assessment.

Wagner, J. L. 1982. A Study of the Impact of Reimbursement Strategies on the Diffusion of Medical Technologies, vols. I and II. Report prepared for the Health Care Financing Administration, Washington, D.C.

Wardell, W., and L. Lasagna. 1975. Regulation and Drug Development. Washington, D.C.: American Enterprise Institute.

Product Liability and Medical Device Regulation: Proposal for Reform

SUSAN BARTLETT FOOTE

The revolution in medical device technology in the last two decades has not occurred in a policy vacuum. This paper focuses on two very different and comprehensive public policies—product liability and regulation—that have emerged in response to the growing availability of medical devices. Congress passed the Medical Device Amendments of 1976 (P.L. 84-295; 90 Stat. 539 [codified at 21 U.S.C. 360c]) to promote the safety of new technological products. Since that time, there has been an increasing number of product liability cases in state courts, including lawsuits against medical device manufacturers.

The goals of product liability are broader than those of regulation, and include compensation of individuals, deterrence of unsafe products, and punishment of socially irresponsible firms. Although both systems reflect deeply held American values, neither has fully achieved its goals. Moreover, medical devices are subject to these two regimens simultaneously; serious distortions have occurred as the two interact. Both systems have been controversial and have generated heated debate, and proposals for reform have proliferated in recent years.

This paper presents an analytical framework from which the strengths and weaknesses of product liability and regulation, as they affect medical devices, can be appraised. The framework is premised on two observations: First, the values underlying product liability and regulation serve both individual and social functions. The primary goal of individuals is to receive compensation for product-related injuries. Plaintiffs initiate lawsuits because they may offer the only source of money to cover expenses related to their injuries. Tort law also has social functions, which include punishment of irresponsible producers and deterrence of future harmful actions. Regulation benefits society by deterring the production or use of unsafe products, mandating disclosure of information, and punishing irresponsible corporations. Much of the dissatisfaction with product liability and regulation as they relate to medical devices arises from inefficient allocation of these individual and social functions.

The second fundamental observation is that medical devices should be distinguished from other consumer products for purposes of policy reform. Medical devices present unique issues, and their special nature led to the passage of medical device legislation. Drugs and devices are the only consumer products subject to intense scrutiny through a federal agency such as the Food and Drug Administration (FDA). (Although there are many similarities between pharmaceuticals and medical devices, it is beyond the scope of this paper to analyze drug issues.)

In addition, medical devices are an integral part of the health care system that provides essential services to the American public. All policies that directly or indirectly affect medical devices must acknowledge their impact on the health care system as a whole. For example, if product liability suits raise the costs of particular products, this result must be evaluated against the public's demands for widespread access to advanced medical technology and the real cost constraints that government and third-party payers face.

Effective policy reform requires an understanding of the individual and social functions underlying product liability and regulation generally, and in relation to medical devices specifically. The framework presented here offers justifications for these fundamental distinctions and sets the stage upon which the specifics of policy reform for medical devices can be debated.

INDIVIDUAL AND SOCIAL FUNCTIONS: THE LIMITS OF REGULATION AND PRODUCT LIABILITY

The primary purpose of federal safety regulation is to deter behavior that unacceptably imperils the general public (Breyer, 1982; Lowrance, 1976). The Medical Device Amendments of 1976 are a classic example of social regulation. Congress authorized the FDA to regulate all medical devices to ensure that these products were safe and efficacious (21 U.S.C. 360c). The law created a three-tiered classification scheme; only devices that pose the most significant safety risks must meet premarket approval standards equivalent to new drugs. However, all medical devices are subject to general controls during production and after the product has entered the stream of commerce. These controls include the federal government's power to order recalls, notification of defects, and repair. Because of the difficulty of uncovering all device-related problems before marketing, the authority to acquire information on medical devices in the marketplace and to respond to newly discovered public health risks is a critical FDA responsibility.

The medical device law has been in place for over a decade. Implementation of the law has not been without controversy: Congress expressed dissatisfaction with FDA's commitment to device regulation in 1983 (U.S. Congress, 1983). Bills to improve the law have been proposed (U.S. Congress, 1986). Although the basic premises of the legislation are sound, problems have arisen because of limited regulatory tools—primarily postmarket surveillance constraints, shifting political philosophies that have led to inconsistent enforcement, insufficient financial resources at FDA, and some cumbersome procedures, particularly in the area of standard-setting.

Unlike the purely social functions of regulation, tort law has a more diverse mandate. Generally defined, tort law encompasses civil wrongs where one person's conduct causes injury to another in violation of a duty imposed by law (Kionka, 1977). The principles of tort law developed within the common law tradition, evolving through state court judicial decisions. In the context of product liability, tort law encompasses both negligence, based on fault, and strict liability, which is premised on no-fault principles (Prosser and Keeton, 1984).

It is generally agreed that tort law has three major functions. A primary goal of every product liability suit is to compensate deserving victims of accidents by awarding compensatory damages. These damages can include economic losses such as medical expenses or lost wages, and noneconomic losses such as pain and suffering. This is tort law's response to individuals.

In addition, tort law seeks to deter socially undesirable conduct. In the context of medical devices, the goal is to prevent the production of unsafe products that cause harm (Sugarman, 1985). This goal benefits society generally, not injured individuals. Implicit in the concept of deterrence are notions of justice. In some instances, tort law punishes individual corporations for socially unacceptable behavior by seeking redress. In a civil system, such punishment occurs through assessment of punitive damages.

Finally, there are traditional economic justifications for tort law; these also benefit society generally. First, resources are allocated efficiently by attributing the social costs of accidents to those who "cause" them—for example, irresponsible corporations. Alternatively, tort law may spread the costs of accidents widely to mitigate the rise in prices that would occur as the costs of harm are internalized (Calabresi, 1970). If the legal system is efficient, both individual and social goals of tort law will be met.

Tort law, however, fails to meet these goals generally, and fails to meet them in relation to medical devices specifically. Admittedly, this conclusion is drawn on what is generally recognized to be limited statistical data (American Bar Association, 1987). Information on product-related injuries is sketchy because injuries may go unreported. Lawsuits may provide additional facts, but over 90 percent of such suits are settled out of court; insurance information on settlements is not public information. Trial court rulings are not generally reported— only appellate opinions are widely available. Although there is some dispute regarding the actual state of affairs in tort law, we do know that insurance rates, the number of cases filed, and the amount of jury awards have all been rising in recent years (Peterson, 1987).

Product liability law has had an impact on medical device users and producers. Improvements in FDA's reporting system have led to increases in notifications of potentially hazardous device-related incidents, although severe underreporting still exists (General Accounting Office, 1986). Recalls of medical devices have been rising as well. Costs of liability suits have been directly responsible for at least one bankruptcy (A. H. Robins Co., producer of the Dalkon Shield), and some firms have left medical device fields because of liability costs, for example anesthesia device producers and vaccine manufacturers (Rordamor, 1984).

Though incomplete, sufficient information exists to draw general conclusions. First, product liability does not compensate victims of accidents fairly or equitably. Studies show that arbitrary factors such as geography (Danzon, 1984), quality of lawyers, and wealth of defendants result in similarly situated plaintiffs receiving very different awards (Fleming and Sugarman, 1980; Sugarman, 1985). A capricious relationship has been shown to exist between the amount plaintiffs' recover and the seriousness of their injuries (Fleming and Sugarman, 1980).

The legal system also exacts a terrible toll on injured people because of long delays between injury and recovery and the risk of no recovery after protracted litigation. Injured people receive lump sums instead of payments as they need them. Sugarman (1985) has argued persuasively that, when plaintiffs are compensated, tort law compensates them in a whimsical, arbitrary fashion, similar in many respects to a lottery.

Compensation of individuals for device-related problems illustrates these general observations. First, similarly situated plaintiffs in mass tort cases—for example, the Dalkon Shield, pacemaker, and toxic shock/tampon suits—received vastly disparate awards. The awards often depended upon when the action was filed and where the case was brought.

Second, producers view the product liability system as unpredictable; it can as easily deter the production of desirable products as discourage undesirable ones (Eads and Reuter, 1983). In the area of health-related products, valuable innovations have been lost or delayed. Critics point to areas of contraceptive research, vaccine development, and anesthesia devices as having been particularly affected by unpredictable liability consequences (Galen, 1986; Rordamor, 1984). Additionally, conflicting rules among the 50 states exacerbate the uncertainty of the liability system. It is no wonder that firms treat liability as "random noise" (Eads and Reuter, 1983).

This is a particular problem under strict liability, which holds a manufacturer liable even in the absence of fault. In *Greenman* v. *Yuba Power Products, Inc.,*[1] the California Supreme Court extended strict liability to product-related injuries for the first time. Applying the principles in a later case, *Barker* v. *Lull Engineering,*[2] courts found products defective if they fail to perform as safely as the user would expect, or if the defendant cannot prove that the benefits of the design outweigh the risks. The *Restatement of Torts,* a compendium of the views of leading legal scholars, recommends limiting application of these principles to products that pose generic risks—so-called "unavoidably unsafe" products[3]—and cites vaccines and drugs as examples of such products. Some state courts have consistently upheld this exception to strict liability; others have not. In *Beshada* v. *Johns-Manville Products Corp.,*[4] the New Jersey Supreme Court held that a state-of-the-art defense is irrelevant for strict liability; manufacturers are responsible for failure to warn of dangers that were undiscoverable at the time of manufacture.

While there continues to be uncertainty among the jurisdictions on this issue (Page, 1983; Schwartz, 1985), there is also uncertainty within certain states. For example, the California appellate courts have been inconsistent in regard to medical devices. In the most recent case involving the drug diethylstilbestrol (DES), *Brown* v. *Superior Court,*[5] the appellate court held that strict liability does not apply to drugs with unexpected side effects. Thus, plaintiffs could only use a theory of negligence to sue the producer. However, in *West* v. *Johnson & Johnson,*[6] a case involving toxic shock syndrome related to the use of tampons, the court allowed the victim to use the "consumer expectation" test derived from the *Barker* v. *Lull Engineering*[2] principles of strict liability. The court did not address the question of whether it is proper to use this test when the danger was unknowable at the time, as the defendant company argued. Nor is there discussion of whether the recommendations of the *Restatement of Torts* might be restricted to drugs and vaccines, and therefore be inapplicable to medical devices. The point, however, is clear: There is uncertainty for medical device producers in the liability system.

In addition to compensating individuals for device-related problems, product liability suits may also seek to punish corporations for egregious behavior through the imposition of punitive damages (Mallor and Roberts, 1980). Studies document a growing tendency to award punitive damages in product liability cases (Peterson, 1987; but see Daniels, 1986). An interesting anomaly occurs, however, because of the mingling of individual and social goals in tort. Litigation involves disputes between an individual and a producer. Traditionally, court awards simply transfer damages, including any punitive damages, from the defendant to the plaintiff. Thus, some plaintiffs receive windfall awards in addition to the monetary damages intended to compensate them fully for their injuries. Critics question the merits of a system that "punishes" a company by conferring these monetary judgments on fully compensated individuals. Punitive damages have been awarded in a number of highly visible device cases: $3 million against an anesthesia device producer (*Airco* v. *Simmons First National Bank*),[7] $1.35 million against a tampon producer (*O'Gilvie* v. *International Playtex*)[8] and several million dollars against A. H. Robins, the producer of the controversial Dalkon Shield (Schwadel, 1985). One can argue that there should be mechanisms to chastise certain producers, yet can question whether this particular tool is efficient or rational.

Finally, there is little dispute that tort law is inefficient. Transaction costs have been described as "fabulously expensive" (Sugarman, 1985). Generally, less than half of the premiums paid for liability insurance go to compensation. The Inter-Agency Task Force on Products Liability estimated that 40 percent of premiums go for underwriting expenses and profit and 20 percent of premiums go for loss-adjustment expenses; this leaves only 40 cents of every premium dollar available to compensate victims (cited in Fleming and Sugarman, [1980]). Economists have argued that these costs should be internalized, and the cost of accidents should be reflected in the price of a product or activity. Products or activities with higher accident rates will therefore be less attractive in the marketplace. But medical devices are part of the health care system and are not part of a free market system. Much of the costs of medical devices will be borne by public payers, private insurers, or employers. Moreover, it is frequently impossible to assign, and therefore internalize, accident costs to a specific product. It has been noted that:

[I]n the case of a dangerous drug, not only would the drug in all likelihood be totally withdrawn from the market after its risks have been discovered but the cost of compensation would in any event probably be spread among all or most other products of the particular manufacturer, with the result that the consumers of the safe drugs would in effect be bearing the accident costs of the dangerous drug. In a theoretical free market, this "externalizing" of the cost might be blocked, but often—and prescription drugs is a good example—such a hypothesis is wholly unrealistic (Fleming and Sugarman, 1980).

Finally, uncertainty costs are a fundamental element of inefficiency. The tort system carries great uncertainty for producers. As Fleming and Sugarman persuasively wrote, tort encourages investment in litigation rather than investment in safety.

DISTORTIONS CAUSED BY INCONSISTENCIES BETWEEN REGULATION AND PRODUCT LIABILITY

Supporters of the present product liability system may argue that, in the absence of alternatives, a flawed compensation system is better than none at all. Justifications for retaining the present liability system, however, weaken in the face of distortions caused by interactions between regulation and product liability. In theory, there is no conflict between the goals of product liability and regulation generally, or in relationship to medical devices specifically. Although their institutional structures and mandates are quite different, both tort and regulation seek to deter the production or use of unsafe products. Tort law has the additional goals of compensation and punishment. In practice, however, the interplay between these two institutional regimens creates tensions that can undermine the success of each.

Every well-intentioned producer wants to make a "safe" product. The conclusion that a particular product is "safe" is a value judgment (Lowrance, 1976). Once the risks of a product are measured, it will be considered "safe" only if the risks are found to be "acceptable" when weighed against the benefits. The problem facing producers is that a regulatory evaluation of safety is very different from a judicial one.

The FDA, as regulator, is concerned with public health; its focus is on broad social policy. Scientists on the agency staff—aided by advisory panels of independent experts—evaluate products prospectively. The agency does have some postmarketing remedies if defects are later uncovered, but these remedies do not involve compensation for harm.

Product liability cases are initiated by individuals whose primary interest is compensation for their injuries. This view is retrospective; the harm already has been incurred. The opportunity for compensation is contingent on a finding that the product is unsafe, and there is enormous pressure for the court to make a finding in order to compensate. It has been noted that "in demanding such explanations, tort lawyers may press scientists beyond their capacity to provide answers" (Abraham and Merrill, 1986). The intensely individual function of product liability is reflected in the nature of the jury system: a jury of one's peers, confronted with an injured individual and a faceless corporation, may press for a conclusion of liability in order to compensate.

Product liability law also requires that the allegedly unsafe product cause the harm. The pressure to compensate an individual encourages judicial decision makers to link the harm and the product, resulting in rules of evidence that substitute "legal sufficiency" for scientific certainty. This was recently illustrated in *Wells* v. *Ortho Pharmaceutical Co.,*[9] in which the court held:

A cause-effect relationship need not be clearly established by animal or epidemiological studies before a doctor can testify that, in his opinion, such a relationship exists. As long as the methodology employed to reach such a conclusion is sound, . . . products liability law does not preclude recovery until a "statistically significant" number of people have been injured or until science has had the time and resources to complete sophisticated laboratory studies of the chemical.

Law turns scientific method on its head. As the *New York Times* editorialized: These "decisions are of great concern to the medical community because they indicate that the courts will not be bound by reasonable scientific standards of proof" (New York Times, December 27, 1986). Deviation from scientific principles also occurs because decisions are made by laypersons—the judge or jurors.

Differences between concepts of regulatory and legal safety are acknowledged by the treatment of regulatory conclusions in court. It is well accepted in most jurisdictions that "mere" compliance with federal or state regulations does not preclude a jury from concluding that the product is unsafe, either because the design is defective or the warnings inadequate (*Ferebee* v. *Chevron*).[10] Courts may draw these conclusions even if the FDA has mandated the precise language in the warning labels and has determined that the product is safe and effective. Even where states have interpreted case law to mean that a medical product that meets FDA requirements is not defective for purposes of strict liability, one trial lawyer asserted that "an effective presentation can be made in court that the FDA's standards for medical devices do not preclude recovery since they are so ineffectual as to be virtually meaningless" (Raney, 1986). Many jurisdictions treat the failure to comply with any FDA requirements as per se negligence. In essence, there are no positive incentives for producers to comply fully with FDA requirements. Compliance provides no protection in a court of law.

In addition, the unpredictable judicial climate undermines the FDA's goal of disclosure of information, particularly once the product has entered the stream of commerce. Although manufacturers are required to report adverse reactions, health care providers report such reactions on a voluntary basis. And information submitted to the FDA is never rewarded; the company faces enormous risks upon reporting. For example, plaintiffs' attorneys often can acquire reported information. Rather than encouraging a free and frequent flow of information, including information that may ultimately prove that a product is not defective, the opposite occurs (General Accounting Office, 1986). While the public should not be foreclosed from access to information on risks, this must be balanced against the need to encourage a free flow of information that can be used to make effective public health policy. Scientific improvements and protection of public health depend upon information; yet, providing such information in a volatile liability environment may be more threatening to producers than would non-compliance with FDA reporting requirements.

This problem is exacerbated by the fact that product liability law does more than merely compensate. In the name of deterrence and punishment, individual plaintiffs may receive windfalls in the form of punitive damages that are intended to serve a social function. But the social goal of information gathering is threatened by pressure from individuals and their lawyers for compensation. These inconsistencies could be reduced if the compensation function now served by tort law were separated from the broader social functions poorly served by inconsistent tort and regulatory principles. In the process, we might develop more efficient mechanisms for meeting both individual and social goals.

MEDICAL DEVICES AS A SPECIAL KIND OF CONSUMER PRODUCT: A FRAMEWORK FOR APPROACHING REFORM

At present, medical device regulation and product liability rules have inefficiently and ineffectively addressed both the individual goal of compensation and the social goals of deterrence and punishment. Realignment of the responsibilities of regulation and product liability will lead to a better fit between the desired goals and the processes by which they can be achieved.

But to accomplish this, medical devices first must be distinguished from other consumer products. There are two compelling reasons to make this distinction. First, medical devices are an integral part of the health care system. Any policies that affect devices ultimately affect health care. As we have seen, imposition of costs on particular products, especially in the inefficient manner provided for by the court system, will raise the prices of these products, classes of products, or products produced by particular firms. Because 40 percent of all medical technology is paid for by the government, higher product prices may conflict with federal efforts at cost-containment. Higher prices also may reduce the availability of desired products and impede their diffusion to all who need them. Ignoring the interface between medical devices and medical care is short-sighted and, in the long run, may reduce innovation and be destructive to values of access and equity.

A second justification for realignment is the presence of the FDA. The regulatory authority of the FDA is clear testimony to the fact that, as a society, we consider devices qualitatively different from other consumer products. For decades, the FDA has played a crucial role in protecting the public health through regulation of drugs and devices. Given its size, expertise, and jurisdiction, reform proposals should take advantage of the FDA's unique potential to protect health and safety.

A number of proposals to change various aspects of regulation and tort have been presented. While some contain interesting features, none address the unique problems of medical devices or acknowledge the importance of both social and individual values inherent in regulation and tort, and the tensions between them.

Although deregulation has been a rallying cry in recent years, no one has seriously called for dismantling FDA regulation and substituting exclusive reliance on tort. If anything, there has been pressure for more and better regulation. FDA received a scathing review of its performance in a congressional report in 1983; the House Report accused FDA of "cavalier disregard for potential consequences" and "bureaucratic neglect for public health and safety that shocks the conscience" (U.S. Congress, 1983).

However, there has been significant activity at both the federal level and among the states to alter product liability rules. Congress has held many hearings on the issue, and a number of bills have been introduced during the 1980s (Foote, 1986). In these proposals, manufacturers of all types of products have sought to limit their liability exposure. Consumer groups have generally opposed these efforts.

Pharmaceutical and medical device manufacturers, however, are subject to FDA requirements designed to protect public health. The Pharmaceutical Manufacturers Association (PMA) and the Health Industry Manufacturers Association have lobbied for provisions that recognize the conflict between regulatory policy and tort. PMA proposed a government standards defense, arguing that the process of premarket approval for new prescription drugs and other regulated products should be an acceptable defense for both compensatory and punitive damages in a tort case (Health Industry Manufacturers Association, 1985; Pharmaceutical Manufacturers Association, 1986). However, these proposals overlook the widely held public belief that people are entitled to compensation for harm, particularly harm caused by negligence. Individual citizens may oppose the trends in tort law without compromising a belief in some form of compensation. And, unlike all other industrialized societies (many of which have more restrictive tort rules), the United States has no comprehensive social insurance net for injured victims other than for workers injured on the job. In the absence of alternative mechanisms to compensate, proposals to limit compensation through the tort system appear self-serving and are politically unrealistic.

Some reformers, recognizing the general limitations of product liability, have proposed comprehensive accident compensation plans similar to those in New Zealand and other Western countries (Sugarman, 1985). These proposals would protect the value of compensation for individual harms and may be feasible. Given the federal deficit, however, the uncertain costs of new widespread compensation programs of this magnitude make them politically impractical. Yet it can be argued that more limited alternatives addressing health care issues may be essential to protect health care delivery, even if only as interim solutions.

Other reformers have proposed substituting private sector initiatives for public solutions, such as trading contract rights to sue (O'Connell, 1984). While these proposals may be intrinsically interesting, there appears to be no significant support for eliminating the government's role as guardian of public health and safety.

It is my view that we need new, creative approaches to medical device policy. The following proposal incorporates the fundamental principle essential to rational reform: Individual and social functions need to be decoupled in a framework that treats medical devices as a special kind of product. Within this boundary, the discussion will identify the areas in which further debate must take place.

Overview of Reform Proposal

Figure 1 illustrates the broad contours of a proposed institutional realignment. First, three stages are described that provide a road map

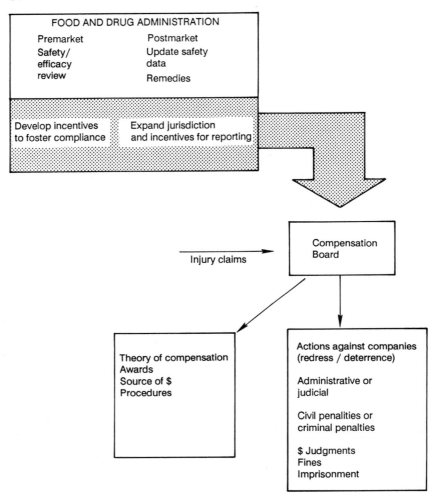

FIGURE 1   Proposed institutional realignment.

for reform. Issues that will need to be resolved in each stage also are identified.

At stage 1, FDA would retain its present premarket and postmarket authority over medical devices. In addition, incentive systems would be developed to foster compliance with FDA regulations and to improve the flow of information to the agency. FDA would thereby retain its important social function of protecting the public health by regulating all medical devices.

Stage 2 creates a new administrative mechanism for compensating individuals harmed by medical devices. A Compensation Board would receive injury claims from individuals. This board would have access to the FDA data and expertise. The purpose of this compensation scheme would be to provide uniform, expeditious, and equitable awards for individuals injured by medical products and to separate compensation of individuals from other social goals.

Stage 3 creates new mechanisms for meeting the social goals of redress and deterrence. Individuals would no longer have the right or the responsibility to redress social grievances through the product liability process. The FDA, the agency entrusted with protecting public health, would bring claims against corporations for corporate behavior determined by law to be socially irresponsible. Like the Securities and Exchange Commission, the FDA would become the watchdog for society at large.

The Stages Described: Issues for Debate

Stage 1

During stage 1, FDA would retain the general contours of its present mandate. However, several reforms could resolve some of the existing tensions within the liability and regulatory systems. New rules would be designed that provide positive incentives (in addition to the negative sanctions) for complying with FDA procedures, both before marketing and after approval. Thus, companies would benefit from fully cooperating with FDA. The public also would benefit from more timely and complete information on medical device hazards. The positive incentive for compliance with FDA during stage 1 would be the creation of a defense to, or a bar against, actions for redress at stage 3. Thus, companies would know that no punitive damage awards or other civil or criminal penalties would be assessed if they comply with the FDA. However, compliance would not prevent injured parties from receiving compensation at stage 2, if all the requirements of that process were met. In summary, rules would be drafted that provide greater certainty to producers, better information, and increased compliance (more safety), with little increased regulatory costs. With greater certainty, liability insurance may be cheaper to purchase, and some companies with conscientious compliance systems might even be willing to self-insure, knowing that their liability would be limited to compensation claims.

One issue to consider at stage 1 is the possibility of extending FDA mandatory reporting requirements to health care providers. While providers are most likely to know of defects in, or problems related to, medical devices, they now are not required to report them to the FDA. The threatening liability environment discussed in relation to manufacturers also applies to physicians and other providers. The absence of good provider data is a weak link in the FDA information bank and is illogical if accurate information is the goal. However, this proposition would involve the federal government even more deeply in decisions of health care providers, and could prove excessively burdensome.

Stage 2

Stage 2 makes a major change in the present compensation process, shifting compensation decisions from the courts—where it is inappropriately imbedded in social policy and burdened with inefficient processes—to an administrative federal agency. The challenge is to create a system that is faster, fairer, and more efficient than the present one. Several major issues need to be resolved.

First, who decides? The Compensation Board must be an expert, independent, and diverse body that would administer the rules credibly. There are many possible models. For example, the Federal Trade Commission (FTC) has established an autonomous body of administrative law judges that have expertise in FTC policy but are independent of FTC policymakers. A similar semi-independent board could be established with access to FDA data and FDA expertise.

The individuals on the Compensation Board could develop expertise over time, as do hearing officers for the Social Security Administration and the FTC, and could be assisted by an advisory board established to review decisions (see Figure 2). There are a number of models for such an advisory board, including the Prospective Payment Assessment Commission, which is a 15-person permanent independent commission with members representing various sectors of the health care industry. FDA itself has significant experience in the management of technical advisory panels that assist in FDA decisions.

The second issue to be resolved is what the Compensation Board's operative theories of compensation will be. Elements of the compensation theory include principles for compensation, types of awards, and sources of funds for these awards. The goal would be to provide some monetary recompense for injuries caused by medical devices. Debate will center on whether the system should be no-fault, like workers compensation, or fault-based, like negligence law. There could be a blending of the principles of compensation with the nature of the awards. For example, if the injury were generic to the product and

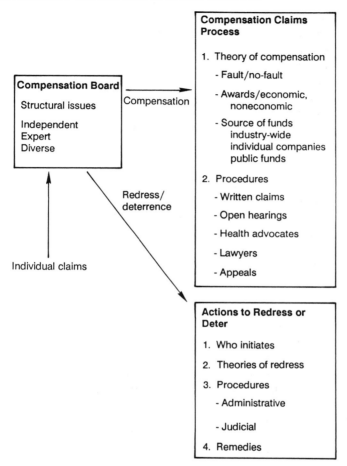

FIGURE 2   Proposed Compensation Board, shifting compensation decisions from the courts to an administrative federal agency.

not based on fault, the award could be for economic losses only (i.e., medical costs, lost wages, etc.), with reductions for medical payments covered by insurance. Under a fault principle, the award could be higher and could include other losses such as pain and suffering. At no point would there be awards for punitive damages in stage 2, because these awards serve a purely social, not an individual, function. It is important to remember that the entire theoretical structure can be designed to balance the goals of compensation with the competing values of access and cost-containment for all individuals.

Development of appropriate theories of compensation and the

procedures to implement these theories would be the most challenging tasks. If the system is fault-based, the language and processes of law inevitably would enter the system. At worst, the tort system would simply be replicated in a new forum. On the other hand, a no-fault system raises the spectre of excessive claims, possibly including efforts to transfer injuries caused by user error (still subject to the tort system) to the product in order to take advantage of the cheaper and more streamlined administrative process. Further work is clearly necessary to resolve these concerns. The success or failure of proposals of this type depends, to a large extent, on careful articulation of the theory of compensation for harm.

The third issue to be resolved concerns the source of funds. There are several alternatives. For example, no-fault awards could be paid from general industry contributions based on assessed fees (size of company, dollar amount of sales, etc.). This would spread the costs of unexpected adverse reactions as widely as possible across the medical devices industry. An alternative would be to establish a public fund, perhaps supplemented with private money, for unintended, unexpected adverse reactions (in effect, a public-private partnership). In either case, individual firms would be responsible for any injuries that are determined by the Compensation Board to be the firm's fault; the board could bill them for awards assessed against them during a given calendar year. Proceeds from any civil liability assessed at stage 3 could be added to the fund and used to defray administrative costs. The Compensation Board would administer the medical device compensation fund, paying successful claimants on a continuing basis rather than with a lump sum, when appropriate.

The final issue to be resolved in stage 2 is the procedures that will be used by the Compensation Board. Claims could be in the form of written petitions or hearings. Written petitions would be cheaper to process than public hearings and may be sufficient for most, if not all, claims. The important point would be to reduce or eliminate legal aspects of the compensation process and concentrate on medical issues. This would be a medical, not a legal, inquiry. Primary data would include the facts of the case; medical records; and sworn affidavits of injured individuals, witnesses, and medical device manufacturers. One could argue that judgments should be based only on scientific principles of cause, but such a requirement may preclude recovery for significant numbers of individuals. Once again, policy trade-offs would be crucial; how much money can or should we commit to these claimants, given the overall impact on the costs and concomitant availability of health care? A system that limited compensation too narrowly would be opposed by consumers; a system that paralleled too closely the tort system would not be an improvement. Unlike the uncertainty of the tort system, however, rules of procedure for the Compensation Board could be carefully developed in advance, balancing the needs of the individual against the impact on corporations and the health care system as a whole.

In developing institutional structures, several critically important issues must be kept in mind. First, the goal is equitable, efficient, fast, and fair compensation. Elimination of unnecessary procedures, development of rules of compensation and schedules for multiple claims, and streamlining and simplifying the process are all important. The overall need is to develop a compensation system that can satisfy the public's need for compensation for harm without compromising the important values of medical device innovation and health care access and distributional equity.

Stage 3

Redress of grievances fulfills a social function. The criminal law system illustrates this point. Victims of crime cannot punish the perpetrators; prosecution and punishment are public functions. Similarly, it can be argued that the FDA, as guardian of the public health, should have an exclusive right of action against companies that deserve additional sanctions beyond compensating injured individuals. This proposal raises several issues: Can the FDA be trusted to bring cases against regulated industries? Agency inaction when action is appropriate would undermine the important goals of deterrence and redress. Although the FDA has not demonstrated such tendencies, implementation of new regulatory tools is always somewhat unpredictable. Various mechanisms could be created to encourage the FDA to take appropriate action. For example, a unanimous Compensation Board recommendation to pursue stage 3 sanctions could automatically trigger them. The commissioner of the FDA, or the secretary of the Department of Health and Human Services, could have the discretion to bring sanctions. Individuals and public interest groups could petition the agency to act; however, they would have no individual right of action.

If a decision were made to pursue redress in a particular case, what actions would be available? Although the FDA has no civil remedies now, several reform proposals in the past have considered conferring this power on the agency. A civil action could be based on allegations that the company had engaged in fraud, misrepresentation, or willful endangerment of the public health. Such an action could generate large monetary fines that could be transferred to the Medical Device Trust Fund and used to defray compensation costs. In addition, the FDA could expand its present criminal sanctions so that individuals within corporations might also receive criminal punishment for wrongful actions, including imprisonment or fines. (There is a significant body of literature that discusses the difficulties in deterring corporate malfeasance and punishing corporate bad actors [Metzger, 1984].)

In general, the FDA would act to defend public health and safety much as the Securities and Exchange Commission acts in the public interest. The social goals of deterrence and redress are most appropriately protected by a public, not a private, entity.

CONCLUSION

There are several important values that undergird the tort system and medical device regulation. The appropriate test for evaluating existing systems is not whether they achieve one goal, such as compensation, but whether they best achieve a combination of goals, including deterrence and redress, compensation, and efficiency. These goals must be achieved within the context of the health care system as a whole, recognizing the additional values of widespread access to care at reasonable cost and support for innovative technology. The framework developed here distinguishes the individual and the social functions of these two systems, realigning them to achieve an efficient process and to facilitate the attainment of the defined goals. This can only be accomplished if medical devices are considered separate from other consumer products and are viewed as an integral part of the health care system. If we do not address the significant limitations of the present tort and regulatory policies in the near future, we may find ourselves making health care compromises that obstruct the values that we intend to protect.

NOTES

[1]59 Cal. 2d 57 (1963).
[2]20 Cal. 3d 413 (1978).
[3]Restatement of the Law, Second, Torts American Law Institute.
[4]447 A. 2d 539 (1982).
[5]227 Cal. Rptr. 768 (1986).
[6]220 Cal. Rptr. 437 (1985).
[7]638 S.W. 2d 600 (1982).
[8]609 F. Supp. 817 (1985).
[9]788 F.2d 741 (11 Cir.) (1986).
[10]736 F.2d 1529 (1984).

BIBLIOGRAPHY

Abraham, K. S., and R. A. Merrill. 1986. Scientific uncertainty and the courts. Issues in Science and Technology II(2):93–107.

American Bar Association. 1987. Report of the Action Commission to Improve the Tort Liability System. Chicago, Ill.: American Bar Association.

Breyer, S. G. 1982. Regulation and Its Reform. Cambridge: Harvard University Press.

Calabresi, G. 1970. The Costs of Accidents. New Haven, Conn.: Yale University Press.

Daniels, S. 1986. Punitive Damages: Storm on the Horizon? Preliminary Report of the Punitive Damages Project, American Bar Foundation. Chicago, Ill.: S. Daniels.

Danzon, P. 1984. The frequency and severity of medical malpractice claims. Journal of Law and Economics 27:115

Eads, G., and P. Reuter. 1983. Designing Safer Products: Corporate Responses to Product Liability Law and Regulation. Santa Monica, Calif.: Rand Institute for Civil Justice.

Fleming, J. G., and S. D. Sugarman. 1980. Perspectives on compensating accident victims. Pp. 175–203 in Compensating for Research Injuries, Report of the President's Commission for the Study of Ethical Problems in Medicine and Biomedical and Behavioral Research. Washington, D.C.: The Commission.

Foote, S. B. 1986. Coexistence, conflict and cooperation: Public policies toward medical devices. Journal of Health Politics, Policy and Law 11:501–523.

Galen, M. 1986. Birth control options limited by litigation. National Law Journal 9(October):1, 26.

General Accounting Office. 1986. Medical Devices: Early Warning of Problems Is Hampered by Severe Underreporting. Washington, D.C.: General Accounting Office.

Health Industry Manufacturers Association. 1985. Memorandum from Legal Task Force of Product Liability (on file with author).

Kionka, E. J. 1977. Torts: Injuries to Persons and Property. St. Paul, Minn.: West Publishing Co.

Lowrance, W. W. 1976. Of Acceptable Risk. Los Altos, Calif.: William Kaufmann, Inc.

Mallor, J., and B. Roberts. 1980. Punitive damages: Toward a principled approach. Hastings Law Journal 31:641.

Metzger, M. B. 1984. Corporate criminal liability for defective products: Policies, problems, and prospects. The Georgetown Law Journal 73:1–88.

New York Times. Editorial. December 27, 1986.

O'Connell, J. 1984. Alternatives to the tort system for personal injury. San Diego Law Review 23:17–35.

Page, J. A. 1983. Generic product risks: The case against comment k and for strict tort liability. New York University Law Review 58:853–891.

Peterson, M. A. 1987. Civil Juries in the 1980's. Santa Monica, Calif.: Rand Institute for Civil Justice.

Pharmaceutical Manufacturers Association. 1986. Tort Reform File (documents on file with author).

Prosser, W., and P. Keeton. 1984. Prosser and Keeton on Torts, 5th ed. St. Paul, Minn.: West Publishing Co.

Raney, M. B. 1986. Medical-device defects. Trial (May):39–42.

Rordamor, W. 1984. Doctor, lawyer, bionics chief. California Lawyer (December):45,101.

Schwadel, F. 1985. Robins and plaintiffs face uncertain future: Chapter 11 filing postpones 5,100 Dalkon Shield cases. Wall Street Journal (August 23):6.

Schwartz, V. E. 1985. Unavoidably unsafe products: Clarifying the meaning and policy behind comment K. Washington and Lee Law Review 42:1139–1148.

Sugarman, S. D. 1985. Doing away with tort law. California Law Review 73:555–664.

U.S. Congress. House of Representatives. 1983. Medical Device Regulation: The FDA's Neglected Child. Report of the Subcommittee on Oversight and Investigations of the Committee on Energy and Commerce, 98th Cong. 1st sess.

U.S. Congress. House of Representatives. H.R. 5516, Introduced September 12, 1986. 99th Cong. 2d sess.

Impact of the Changing Medical Payment System on Technological Innovation and Utilization

STUART H. ALTMAN

When Medicare legislation was drafted in 1965, legislators were determined to control health care costs. Not unreasonably, they decided that the best way to control federal spending on health care was to pay only for the cost of the care that was provided. Legislators reasoned that there are only a few ways in which a particular illness can be treated; if hospitals are paid only for services rendered, they will not make profits from Medicare and costs will be contained.

Since 1965, however, hundreds of analyses and documents have been prepared demonstrating that cost-based reimbursement had the opposite effect. It created a set of economic incentives that rewarded spending and penalized attempts by hospital managers to provide medical care at lower cost. Annual health care spending rose from about 5.5 percent of our gross national product before Medicare was enacted to more than 11 percent in 1987. Some of this additional spending may indeed be beneficial, but there are also many examples of questionable health care expenditures.

For the past 10 years, health care economists and others have warned policymakers, medical practitioners, and the public that the U.S. health care system could collapse if such spending increases continued. Well, the system has not collapsed, but it continues to prosper at the expense of other needed federal services, such as mental health care and guaranteed incomes for the poor. Our gross national product represents the total capacity of our country to purchase needed goods and services. When we double the amount spent on health care, there are fewer resources available for other needs. Although there is no magic number that represents an appropriate amount for the United States to spend for health care services, the question of economic and social trade-offs remains important.

PROSPECTIVE PAYMENT SYSTEM

Congress debated the issue of how to control spending on health care throughout the 1970s without a significant change in the way hospitals were reimbursed by the federal government. In 1982, however, Congress made a fundamental change in the hospital payment system for Medicare. It created the Prospective Payment System (PPS). PPS was heralded by its supporters as a system that would put in place incentives that would make hospitals more cost efficient, a change that was long overdue. On the other hand, some individuals were concerned that there would be problems with PPS. For example, critics feared that many hospitals would go bankrupt and patients would be asked to leave hospitals while they were still in need of care.

Before 1982, Medicare paid for hospital services based on the actual cost of providing that care to Medicare patients. As such, costs varied from hospital to hospital, even for patients being treated for the same illness. PPS changed this by removing the direct link between cost and payment. Under PPS, the payment for each hospital patient is based on the categorization of the patient's illness into one of 468 diagnosis-related groups (DRGs). After a 1-year phase-in, the payment amount for each DRG reflects the average cost of treating patients in that category throughout the United States. Hospital payments do vary, however, to reflect their wage area, the extent to which they are a teaching hospital, whether they are in an urban or rural area, and whether they provided a disproportionate amount of care to low-income patients.

As part of the PPS legislation Congress created the Prospective Payment Commission (ProPAC) to advise it and the executive branch on how to make PPS responsive to changing health care technologies and procedures. The Office of Technology Assessment is responsible for selecting 17 individuals representing various groups involved in the health care system to serve on the commission. I was selected to be its chairman. ProPAC began operation in 1984. Since its inception, it has devoted a major portion of its time and all the time of its 25 staff members to developing an appropriate pricing system for about a dozen new technologies and medical procedures which have become accepted in our medical system. In this paper, I will briefly review the issues surrounding three of these technologies.

Economists have been very successful in teaching those involved in public policy decision-making processes two fundamental lessons: (1) economic resources are finite and (2) economic incentives matter.

It is time that policymakers learn two more economic principles. The first is the concept of elasticity of supply and demand. For example, if the revenue of a product to the manufacturer is reduced (holding the cost of production constant), there is an incentive for manufacturers to produce less of that product—but how much less? The larger the elasticity of supply, the greater will be the reduction in output. Similarly, we know that if the price of a product to the consumer increases, there is a tendency to buy less of that product—but how much less? What is the elasticity of demand?

When we suggest that there are incentives under PPS to use less health care technology, such a statement says nothing about how strong such incentives are and whether they operate across all hospitals. Unfortunately, we almost never talk about the strength of the incentives or the degree of response, which is the elasticity of supply.

The second economic principle concerns income and substitution effects. We know that when the price of a good changes, there is likely to be a change in the quantity consumed. When the price goes up, people usually use less of the good, and when it goes down, people, on average, use more. This is the substitution effect. On the other hand, when the price of a good goes up but one's income also goes up, one might ultimately use more of that good. Despite an incentive to use less of a more expensive good, increased wealth generates an opposing incentive to buy more. This is the income effect.

These principles apply to the hospital industry under PPS. Under the previous cost-based system, a hospital was reimbursed for whatever services it used on a patient. PPS, however, increased the cost of using new medical technology because hospitals faced a fixed budget per patient. Once a DRG category has been established and per-patient reimbursement decided, any extra service or use of an additional test or procedure adds to the cost of treatment but not to the hospital's revenue. Many analysts initially believed that the negative impact of the changed reimbursement system on the purchase and use of medical technologies would be severe. That is, the substitution effect would operate to reduce the acquisition and use of new medical technologies in hospitals.

However, during the first few years of PPS, there have been substantial increases in hospital revenues, which may have made it possible for hospitals to purchase more technology—not less. It is as yet uncertain what the cumulative impact of PPS will be on the purchase and use of medical technologies. In economic terms, will the positive income effect overpower the negative substitution effect?

New Incentives Under the Prospective Payment System

Under PPS, hospitals are paid a fixed payment per diagnosis, and that payment is known beforehand. Therefore, there is an incentive for hospitals to minimize the costs of treatment, including the use of expensive new medical technologies. But the existence of such an incentive does not mean that patients will not receive needed services or that new medical technologies will not be used. Instead, it means that there is some tendency for hospitals to act in that direction.

Often, we hear concerns that the health care system should not cut back too much on those technologies that improve quality of life or the outcome of a medical intervention while adding to health care costs. Congress, too, had similar concerns and instructed ProPAC to advise it on how to introduce new medical technologies into the PPS pricing system. But the technology issue is more complicated and needs more sophisticated analysis than simply saying PPS increases the price of new technology and, therefore, much less technology will be used. For example, there is another incentive that operates in the opposite direction. PPS provides a powerful incentive for hospitals to seek more admissions. The best way to get more admissions is to have doctors who are willing to admit patients to that hospital. The best way to encourage doctors to admit patients to a particular hospital is to make sure that the hospital is up-to-date and has the latest technologies and equipment.

MEDICAL TECHNOLOGIES, HEALTH CARE COSTS, AND THE ROLE OF ProPAC

In 1977, under the auspices of the Robert Wood Johnson Foundation, a conference was held in Sun Valley, Idaho, to look at the impact of medical technology on health care costs. Participants concluded that no one knew. We could document several areas where technology had clearly increased costs. But among the cost-increasing technologies, it was unclear whether technologies with the largest acquisition and operating costs were really the biggest culprits. There were also examples of technologies that had led to substantial reductions in medical costs. When the positive and negative examples were summed, the total impact was unclear.

This finding went against the prevailing wisdom that said we could control escalating health care costs by limiting the use of expensive technologies. Although the evidence did not support it, the general impression in most public policy forums remained that medical technology was overused in the United States and that tough planning and certificate-of-need legislation was needed to control its use. This assumption led to considerable efforts by state and federal planners to limit the availability of a then emerging, new, and expensive technology, computerized tomographic scanners (CTS), and other expensive technologies as well.

It is possible to classify medical technologies into one of four categories. The first type is one that reduces costs and improves the quality of medical care. The pressure to expand the use of these technologies under PPS is substantial.

The second type of technology is one that increases costs to the hospital but reduces costs to the health care system. These technologies are troubling under PPS because the DRG system applies only to hospital care. For example, rehabilitative technologies can result in patients feeling better quicker and, therefore, getting back to work faster. But hospitals which use these technologies only see more costs and no added revenue.

The third type of technology is one that increases costs to the hospital and the health care system, but also increases the quality of medical care. Here the question is whether the added quality justifies the added costs.

Finally, there are those technologies that increase cost but affect quality in only a limited way. Some critics would further argue that there are medical technologies that increase costs and decrease quality. I would like to believe that, over time, such technologies are eliminated by the medical profession itself. But there are knowledgeable people who believe that this is not the case and that a significant amount of money is spent each year on useless and harmful technologies. In any case, there can be no serious objection to a substantial reduction in the use of such technologies.

For ProPAC, the major concern is to focus on the second two types of technologies: those that increase costs to the hospital but decrease costs to the system, and those that increase both costs and quality.

ProPAC commissioners spend much time worrying about these technologies. In general, the commission wants the price system under PPS to be neutral: The payment amount should neither retard the introduction of beneficial technologies nor promote their overuse.

Three new medical technologies that ProPAC has reviewed or is currently studying are cardiac pacemakers, magnetic resonance imaging, and penile prostheses.

Cardiac Pacemakers

There are several types of cardiac pacemakers. Some have one chamber and are relatively simple to operate. In previous years, these single-chamber devices were not as expensive as the dual-chamber, programmable pacemakers that are now available. Unfortunately, the DRG system does not recognize differences in price among the various types of pacemakers; reimbursement is the same regardless of the type of device implanted.

Led by the pacemaker industry, ProPAC was educated to this issue and reviewed PPS reimbursement for this technology. The alternatives are few. If each device is priced differentially by the reimbursement system, then Medicare is returning to cost-based reimbursement, and that is what DRGs were supposed to stop.

The current system, however, is blind to the differences in costs associated with different types of devices. Further, although it costs the hospital more to implant a more expensive device, it does not cost the physician more. Quite the opposite. The physician receives more money for implanting the more complicated device; the physician's incentives may, therefore, be opposed to those of the hospital. What kinds of incentives does that set up? To the extent that the hospitals face an incentive to implant the least expensive device that will produce a desired medical result, that is to be preferred. But what if the incentive is so strong that hospitals implant devices which produce inferior results?

The commission has been very concerned about this potential and decided that the PPS reimbursement approach for pacemakers was not correct. In 1986 ProPAC recommended that there be different payments for single-chamber and dual-chamber devices since these were two distinct technologies and PPS should reimburse them at different rates. The Health Care Financing Administration (HCFA), however, did not go along with this recommendation.

In 1987 the commission again looked at the evidence and found that reimbursement for pacemakers under PPS has become even more complicated. The distinction between single- and dual-chamber devices now appears to be less meaningful: There are more expensive single-chamber devices and cheaper dual-chamber devices. There is actually more price variation within the two pacemaker types than between them. Also, evidence suggests that the current reimbursement system has not yet had a major impact on the type of pacemaker chosen by physicians. Therefore, the commission rescinded its 1986 recommendation and decided to continue to study the issue of appropriate reimbursement for pacemakers.

Magnetic Resonance Imaging

Another issue ProPAC is currently examining is how to pay for the operating costs of magnetic resonance imaging (MRI). After considerable study, HCFA decided that MRI is a useful medical technology. The next question HCFA faced was how to reimburse MRI use under PPS. Under the current system, the purchase price of this new technology is paid for by a capital-cost pass-through. But there is no reimbursement for the higher operating costs of this procedure.

MRI scans are used as a diagnostic test for many different diseases, so it is not possible to establish a separate DRG category for MRI. Fortunately for manufacturers of MRI equipment and for many patients, an MRI scan is often performed as an outpatient procedure and is reimbursable under different rules. But there are Medicare patients who must be hospitalized and who need an MRI scan. For those patients, the hospital receives no additional payment above the applicable DRG rate if an MRI scan is performed.

Again, ProPAC believes that it is inappropriate to introduce a valuable new technology and not develop a mechanism to reimburse hospitals for that technology's operating expenses. ProPAC's goal is neither to encourage the use of MRI nor to discourage its availability and use.

To achieve their goal and to develop a better understanding of the uses and economics of this technology, ProPAC recommended that there be a temporary add-on payment each time an MRI imager is used. The add-on amount ProPAC proposed was modest and was based on what the reimbursement level should be if imagers are being used at their most efficient level.

ProPAC's proposal violated some basic tenets of the DRG system: ProPAC recommended that the payment system be related to the use of a medical device and not a fixed amount per diagnosis. But the commission faced a difficult choice. If it did nothing, this technology would not get paid for and may become underused, particularly if in the future capital expenditures also are included in the DRG payment. Although ProPAC recommended in 1986 and again in 1987 that HCFA develop an MRI add-on for a 3-year period, HCFA and the Congress have not yet accepted this recommendation.

Penile Prostheses

The third technology or device I will discuss is an appropriate payment system for a new type of penile prosthesis. Again, the implanting of penile prostheses is a procedure for which there is one payment amount regardless of the type of device used on the patient. A new type of prosthesis is now available that apparently works much better but costs more than the old one. The prospective payment system does not fully recognize that change in the technology and pays a weighted average of the costs of the various devices that are available. A number of urologists have petitioned ProPAC claiming that the present PPS payment is preventing their patients from receiving what they (the physicians) and their patients believe is the correct treatment.

Just as with cardiac pacemakers, a Medicare patient cannot go to a hospital and request the more expensive device and offer to supplement the government's reimbursement. Only patients who do not accept any Medicare reimbursement can select the technology of their choice. However, they must pay the total hospital bill. Patients who are not wealthy must accept the technology that the hospital and their doctor determine is appropriate.

There are those who say that if PPS becomes even more restrictive, we will see increasing limitations on what Medicare will pay. This will be followed by added pressure to allow patients to supplement the basic reimbursement. Others voice concern about creating a two-class Medicare program in which poorer patients must accept the treatment dictated by Medicare and wealthier patients can choose to supplement that treatment. If no supplementation is allowed and PPS does become more restrictive, then the technological issues reviewed in these three examples will become increasingly important.

IMPACT OF PPS ON MEDICAL TECHNOLOGY

ProPAC believes that the DRG system needs to be more responsive to new medical technology or there will be inappropriate reductions in the use of these services. But to make this case, the commission needs to show the negative effects of the existing DRG system on development and use of medical technologies. What impact or leverage has medical care reimbursement under PPS had on the use, and ultimate manufacture, of new medical technologies? Unfortunately, we still know very little about what has happened. Prospective payment for Medicare was introduced in 1983, and by 1987 we had just begun to understand what happened in 1983–1984.

Although there have been financial problems for some hospitals, particularly rural hospitals, the overall American hospital system appears to have adjusted well to the introduction of PPS. To determine how well hospitals have fared under PPS, ProPAC reviewed changes in hospital revenues and expenses since DRGs were put in place. From

TABLE 1   Change (in percent) in Hospital Expenses, 1976–1986,
Adjusted by the Consumer Price Index (in percent)

Year	Total Expenses	Total Expenses per Capita	Inpatient Expenses	Inpatient Expenses per: Capita	Admission
1976	12.6	11.5	12.2	11.1	8.6
1977	8.6	7.5	8.2	7.1	5.5
1978	4.8	3.7	4.3	3.2	3.9
1979	1.9	0.8	1.8	0.7	−0.8
1980	3.0	1.8	2.9	1.6	0.0
1981	7.6	6.5	7.2	6.2	6.3
1982	9.1	8.1	8.9	7.8	8.8
Average increase, 1976–1982	6.8	5.7	6.5	5.4	4.6
1983	6.8	5.8	6.1	5.1	6.7
1984	0.6	−0.4	−0.7	−1.6	3.1
1985	2.7	1.8	0.5	−0.4	5.7
1986[a]	7.0	6.2	5.1	4.2	7.7
Average increase, 1983–1986	3.5	2.5	1.6	0.7	5.5

[a]Estimate based on the first 8 months of 1986 compared to the first 8 months of 1985.
SOURCE: American Hospital Association National Panel Survey.

1976 to 1982, inpatient expenses, after adjusting for overall inflation, went up 6.5 percent (Table 1) and hospital inpatient revenues went up by an average annual rate of 7.1 percent (Table 2). Under cost-based reimbursement before PPS, therefore, hospital revenues per admission were increasing about 9 percent faster than expenses.

During 1983, the first year of PPS, both revenues and expenses grew by approximately 7.0 percent. But in 1984, inpatient expenses increased 3.1 percent and inpatient revenues grew by 4.2 percent. Two facts about 1984 are important. First, there was a substantial drop in both hospital revenues and expenses. But, more important, hospital revenues increased more rapidly than expenses. That was the year when hospital administrators refrained from purchasing new medical technologies and forced price concessions from hospital suppliers, expecting a tight limit on their revenues.

But hospitals found that reimbursement revenues from Medicare did not fall nearly as fast as they had expected. In fact, during the first year of PPS, actual per-admission costs per Medicare patient were 14.8 percent lower than Medicare revenues. This is a substantial difference, considering that each 1 percent difference is equal to $400 million. Before PPS, Medicare revenues and costs were increasing at

TABLE 2   Change (in percent) in Hospital Revenues, 1976–1986, Adjusted by the Consumer Price Index

Year	Total Revenues	Inpatient Revenues	Outpatient Revenues	Other Revenues	Revenues per: Inpatient Admission	Outpatient Visit
1976	13.6	13.9	17.2	−0.1	10.2	13.5
1977	9.2	9.2	12.8	0.3	6.4	6.3
1978	4.7	4.0	8.2	8.9	3.6	7.7
1979	2.3	2.1	3.0	5.4	−0.6	3.4
1980	3.7	3.7	5.1	−0.4	0.9	2.0
1981	7.7	7.1	9.5	13.3	6.3	8.0
1982	9.6	9.5	11.3	6.7	9.5	10.1
Average increase, 1976–1982	7.3	7.1	9.6	4.9	5.2	7.3
1983	6.8	6.4	11.0	2.2	7.0	8.0
1984	1.7	0.3	9.3	3.8	4.2	7.8
1985	2.4	0.0	14.3	8.5	5.1	9.3
1986[a]	5.8	3.7	15.4	7.9	6.4	6.7
Average increase, 1983–1986	4.2	2.6	12.5	5.6	5.7	8.0

[a]Estimate based on the first 8 months of 1986 compared to the first 8 months of 1985.
SOURCE: American Hospital Association National Panel Survey.

about the same rate. According to the Congressional Budget Office, these higher-than-expected "margins"—i.e., revenues minus costs—will generate $27 billion in excess hospital revenues over 5 years, or approximately $5 billion in excess revenues per year.

When we examine the effect of PPS on specific medical technologies, we find that the use of higher-cost pacemakers has been growing faster than the use of their less expensive counterparts by a margin of four to one, a phenomenon many would not have expected when PPS was introduced. When we look at the newer, more expensive penile prosthesis, the same thing is happening. And MRIs are being purchased by hospitals almost as rapidly as one would have expected before PPS. Even though Medicare is not providing larger reimbursements to hospitals for use of higher-cost devices—and incentives therefore remain to use lower-cost technologies—the introduction and use of expensive new medical technologies appears to be continuing to grow.

Why has this happened? Is it because economic incentives do not matter? I do not think so. I believe it is because of the high Medicare per patient margins earned. For hospitals, the income effect (i.e., larger than expected Medicare revenues) appears to have swamped the substitution effect. Can we be sure this will continue to happen in the future? I am not optimistic. Congress will not allow such high margins as profits to continue to accrue; our nation's budget problems are too pressing.

CONCLUSIONS

I believe that the PPS has much merit and that for most illnesses an average payment amount per DRG is appropriate. But there are situations such as the three technologies I discussed in this paper where an average national rate per diagnosis should not be followed. Instead, I believe we should use a blended reimbursement rate—somewhere between a patient-specific amount and one which relies on a national rate. In so doing, we will take into account somewhat the special needs of each patient.

How fiscally hard do you have to hit a hospital to make the point that they ought to think twice about purchasing and using an expensive new technology? Does the penalty have to be 100 percent, or can it be 25 percent? Economists deal on the margin. We complained for years that cost-based reimbursement generated the wrong incentives by paying for all the added costs of treating a patient with a more expensive procedure. Now, I believe that PPS also generates the wrong incentives by paying for none of the extra expense of using an expensive procedure.

We may have to wait several years before finding out whether the incentives under PPS are as strong as I suggest. My own view is that they ultimately will be shown to be too strong.

A Conflict: Medical Innovation, Access and Cost Containment

SEYMOUR PERRY AND FLORA CHU

Technology is both praised for improving medical care and blamed for contributing to the current problems of the health care system. Technological innovation has enhanced life expectancy, access to care, and health status. At the same time, however, these gains have exacted a substantial price in economic terms. Real per capita health care expenditures rose an average of 4.6 percent and hospital expenses experienced a 5.4 percent increase in real growth from 1973 to 1983, to the mounting concern of policymakers (Merrill and Wasserman, 1985). Though there are other important contributing factors, medical technology has been implicated in from 30 percent (Office of Technology Assessment, 1985a) to 50 percent (Ruby et al., 1985) of this increase.

The medical device industry has produced more than 1,700 different devices (General Accounting Office, 1986), many of them expensive. These devices give physicians tools to improve patient care through life-saving therapy, intensive monitoring, relief of pain, and amelioration of disability. Because modern medical technologies tend to be expensive, however, conflict arises between the desire of policymakers to reduce health care expenditures and the demand for medical technology by health care providers and the public.

Early medical devices were frequently unwieldy and cumbersome, but modern devices are often compact and more versatile. New models of existing devices often expand the useful range of diagnosis or treatment and are superior in durability, reliability in performance, and convenience in application. For example, in 1957 the original cardiac pacemaker weighed 12 pounds and had to be strapped onto the patient, much like a backpack. During the succeeding 30 years, experimentation and development led to important improvements and a broadened range of therapeutic applications. Today the pacemaker weighs 1.5 ounces and is implantable and programmable. It can be designed to treat both rapid and slow cardiac arrhythmias and can control either one or two chambers of the heart (Bessey, 1986).

Yet the "reign of technology" in medicine is also viewed with suspicion (Reiser, 1978). The potential of new medical technologies to produce unintentional harm, their substitution for personal care, and their failure to produce a "magic cure" for the chronic ills of modern society have led observers to challenge the worth of these technologies (Moloney and Rogers, 1979). Furthermore, some medical technologies add to the inflationary rise in health care costs without adding appreciable benefit (Bunker and Schaffarzick, 1986).

Few new medical devices are likely to cost less per unit than the devices they supplant, at least in the short run. New devices tend to be more complex and sophisticated and to entail considerable costs for research and development; when introduced into the health care system, they usually increase costs (Hillman, 1986). Developing the physician's skills in interpreting and refining clinical applications of new devices generates additional costs. Traditionally, new medical devices—as yet unproven—are often employed in tandem with existing technologies with which the physician is familiar. Until their effectiveness and performance in relation to competing technologies are established, the long-term cost-saving potential of new technologies is difficult to ascertain (Steinberg et al., 1985).

In recent years, critics have increasingly decried the health care provider's reliance on therapeutic and rehabilitative technologies and advocate greater efforts in preventive medicine. Although a better lifestyle, proper diet, and regular exercise are laudable goals, it is important to recognize that there are no effective preventive measures currently available for the chronic and degenerative diseases of modern society. Until such measures become available, health care practitioners will have to rely on technological innovations in diagnosis and treatment.

INCENTIVES AND DISINCENTIVES FOR MEDICAL DEVICE INNOVATION

In the years since World War II, the medical device industry has made remarkable contributions to medical progress. Among the technologies developed during the past two decades are computed tomography (CT), magnetic resonance imaging (MRI), hemodialysis systems, artificial joints, fiber-optic endoscopy, and intraocular lenses (Roe, 1985). This technological progress has been enhanced by reliance on cost- and charge-based health care reimbursement and its bias toward medical technology. From 1958 to 1983, sales of medical devices increased from $1 billion to $17 billion (White, 1985). However, the open-ended era of health care reimbursement is drawing to a close. The medical device industry has become acutely sensitive to the marketplace and faces unprecedented uncertainties in the current push to contain health care costs.

The Prospective Payment System

Medicare's Prospective Payment System (PPS), enacted in 1983, established a set of diagnosis-related group (DRG) categories for hospitalized Medicare beneficiaries and payment rates to hospitals based on those categories. Under PPS, hospitals have strong incentives to provide the least resource-intensive treatment. This may lead them to decrease the provision of inpatient services, change the mix of hospital services toward those that are more profitable, and increase specialization to take advantage of savings associated with higher service volumes (Office of Technology Assessment, 1985b).

Since payment is fixed per case, hospital administrators may prefer technologies that produce short-term over long-term savings. Hospital administrators may shy away from adopting some new technologies because of initial capital and start-up costs and uncertainty about their value in patient care. They also may shift care to outpatient settings, thus escaping the cost controls of the DRG payment system. There is evidence that all of the foregoing are happening to at least some extent (General Accounting Office, 1985; Iglehart, 1986).

Medical devices are at a disadvantage in PPS since, with few exceptions, they have not been identified or specified in the construction of DRG categories (Office of Technology Assessment, 1984). Reimbursement associated with the use of implantable devices, such as pacemakers, generally fall under surgical DRG categories, but services using medical devices that do not require surgical intervention, such as gastroscopy or diagnostic imaging, are not independently specified in the DRG reimbursement structure (Bunker and Schaffarzick, 1986).

Incentives embodied in the PPS could stifle innovation of costly medical technologies even if they prove beneficial, but PPS may also lead providers to avoid ineffective, unsafe, or wasteful technologies and may induce innovators and manufacturers to focus on true "breakthrough" and cost-effective technologies (Office of Technology Assessment, 1985b).

The overall level of hospital payments under PPS is probably more important in determining the level of future technological innovation than specific DRG classifications and rates. Historically, the intensity of medical care, which includes increased use of existing services and introduction of new technologies, has risen 4 to 5 percent each year (Anderson and Steinberg, 1984). However, total payment increases under the PPS have thus far been substantially less, ranging from 1 to 2 percent per year. Adoption and use of new medical technologies must be accommodated within the overall operating margin of the hospital. Recent evidence indicates that this margin has been surprisingly large under PPS (Prospective Payment Assessment Commission, 1987). However, operating funds are not specifically set aside for investing in technological change. They may be used for alternative and pressing needs, such as covering the costs of uncompensated care and of cases that cost more than the DRG reimbursement, particularly at rural and public institutions.

The Health Care Finance Administration Decision-Making Process

In the Medicare program, the use of a new technology may first surface when a question about its coverage status arises in the submission of a claim for reimbursement or because of inquiries from providers and manufacturers. Intermediaries may detect the use of a new technology when a claim form is submitted with unrecognizable codes, no codes, or excessive fees for known, established procedures within which the charge for a new technology may be hidden (Bunker et al., 1982).

Medicare contractors generally decide most coverage questions locally. Coverage issues of national interest are referred to the Health Care Finance Administration's (HCFA's) Office of Coverage Policy. If the central office requires medical input to reach a decision, the issue may be placed before the Physician's Panel, made up of representatives from HCFA and the Public Health Service. This panel may then request a formal technology assessment and recommendation from the Office of Health Technology Assessment of the National Center for Health Services Research and Health Care Technology Assessment. HCFA then uses this information to make the final coverage policy decision and notifies Medicare contractors, state Medicaid agencies, and providers.

However, Medicare contractors across the country vary in their implementation of HCFA policy transmittals (Roe et al., 1986; Ruby et al., 1985). This lack of uniformity has been attributed to such factors as the absence of a requirement for legally binding compliance with national coverage policy, insufficient information about specific technologies, and difficulties in understanding HCFA's coverage instructions (Office of Technology Assessment, 1984; Ruby et al., 1985).

A review of technology assessments performed for Medicare and Blue Cross-Blue Shield plans revealed that such assessments were "highly subjective . . . and serve as complements to—rather than substitutes for—scientific evaluations" (Finkelstein et al., 1984). Technology assessments were based on input from published reports and recommendations of government agencies, medical advisory boards, and medical specialty societies. If data on safety and effectiveness were very convincing, then a technology was usually recommended for coverage. Recently, emphasis on cost control has expanded the scope of reimbursement decision-making processes to include questions of cost and cost-effectiveness (Ruby et al., 1985), although in practice consideration of cost-effectiveness remains limited.

Under Medicare's PPS, a decision to cover the costs of a new device or technology marks only the beginning of the process of accommodating that device or technology within the hospital. A new technology must also be assigned to a DRG that is clinically coherent and promotes homogeneity of resource consumption. This centralized assignment process considers the costs of the new technology, available alternate treatment methods, and the administrative aspects of a DRG price adjustment. Conflicts and delays can, therefore, arise between deciding on the appropriateness of covering a particular new medical technology and determining a payment for that health service (Roe et al., 1986). The Prospective Payment Assessment Commission (ProPAC) has been charged with responsibility for advising the Department of Health and Human Services on updating the DRG system, with one of its stated priorities being to facilitate innovation and assure that beneficial technologies are accommodated in the health care delivery system (Prospective Payment Assessment Commission, 1985).

Innovation Under Alternative Health Care Delivery Systems

Under alternative health care delivery systems, such as the managed care approaches in health maintenance organizations and the price competitive models of preferred provider organizations, incentives are to delay coverage or acquisition of major new technologies until adoption is justified on the basis of cost savings or high-volume use. Instead of the short-term savings incentives embodied in the PPS, these providers emphasize long-term cost-effectiveness in selecting new medical devices and technologies. Technologies for use in the ambulatory and home settings will also be highly desirable.

The trend toward investor-owned health care enterprises, entrepreneurship, and corporatization of medicine stresses the "bottom line" and the profit potential of new technologies as well as exploitation of the profitability of existing technologies. For-profit hospitals tend to be newer and more capital-intensive than not-for-profit facilities (Institute of Medicine, 1986) and may promote state-of-the-art technology as a marketing tool. However, technologies that are relevant to the needs of less profitable patients or are inadequately reimbursed will fare less well under these conditions.

The growing clout of large employers who self-insure their workers also adds to a cautionary attitude toward adoption of costly new technology. Increasingly, businesses employ utilization review mechanisms to monitor the use of health care technology by their providers. They are also negotiating contracts with providers on the basis of price and service packages to control health care expenditures for their employees and retirees (Fruen and DiPrete, 1986).

Another recent development has been the increasing monetarization of medicine (Ginzberg, 1984), impinging on the unique, historical relationship between the physician and patient. Increased entrepreneurism, intense competition, and commercialization of medical care have influenced physicians' practice styles and economic self-interests. Under cost-based reimbursement, the physician could deliberately or inadvertently increase the intensity of health care services to the patient, and there were few disincentives to exceed optimal care (Myers and Schroeder, 1981). Now, realities of cost containment and competition have introduced the physician to a greater awareness of—and in some cases a liability for—the economic consequences of prescribed medical care.

Hospitals and alternative health care delivery systems are increasingly monitoring physicians' patterns of care, pressuring them to limit hospital stays and modify treatment procedures, or offering physicians ownership interests or financial incentives to enhance institutional revenues. These arrangements seek to align the economic motives of the physician with those of the institution (Institute of Medicine, 1986). Medical centers, businesses, and multihospital systems have also entered into employment or contractual agreements with physicians, potentially reducing the dominance of the physician's role in deciding appropriate patient care.

The ultimate resolution of this "double agent" role in which the physician is placed in the position of acting both for the patient and for a business institution is uncertain (Relman, 1985). The resultant impact on the use of technology is also unclear at present. Physicians may assert their fiduciary responsibility to provide cost-conscious patient care that is conservative of health care resources. They may increasingly practice according to set protocols, minimizing variability by using formal decision analyses to make complex choices among alternate health care technologies (Detsky, 1987). Rigid standardization of practice styles could encroach upon individuality of care and dampen the drive for innovation in medical care. On the other hand, formal decision making in patient care may be more responsive to profit-making objectives, inducing preferential use of innovative medical technologies that also promote the self-interest of the provider.

FUTURE DIRECTIONS

What does the future promise for technological innovation in medical care? Undoubtedly, cost-containment pressures will continue to dominate the health care system and shape incentives for innovation. The purchasers of care, particularly large employers, will increasingly seek to dictate the benefit mix, to control prices and use, and to determine the settings where services are provided. Managed care—such as health maintenance organizations and preferred provider organizations—and strict utilization review will continue to increase (Fruen and DiPrete, 1986). Competition in health care delivery will intensify as the surplus of physicians and excess capacity of hospitals increases. This may induce providers to differentiate among their products on the basis of price, amenities, and quality.

In response to these pressures, providers and purchasers of care will continue to channel demand for medical devices toward cost-saving innovations. Hospitals will increasingly employ strategies to reduce costs. These may include negotiating bulk purchase orders or preferred buying contracts through multihospital chain arrangements, demanding trial periods or other inducements from device manufacturers in return for future purchase orders, and delaying investments in new medical technologies until clinical and economic benefits are certain. Technologies that enable health care procedures to be performed outside hospitals, speed recovery after surgery, reduce delays between diagnostic testing and medical treatment, and minimize risks of infection and other complications will all be sought. Current examples of such technologies include extracorporeal shock wave lithotripsy for the removal of kidney stones, laser techniques in a variety of applications, and arthroscopic and endoscopic diagnostic and surgical procedures.

Medical device manufacturers face prospects of considerable delays in reimbursement decisions, uncertainty of payment rates, and constraints on hospitals for major acquisitions. For example, magnetic resonance imaging was first introduced to the United States in December 1980, but Medicare coverage was not provided until November 1985. Such lengthy delays may serve to reduce health care costs in the short term by preventing expenditures for device acquisition, but may also make effective technologies unavailable to patient populations that could benefit from them, and may reduce the policy options than can be used to manage the introduction of new technologies (Hillman, 1986).

An increasing emphasis on short-term, cost-reducing technologies may diminish the commitment of medical device manufacturers to initiate long-range projects with uncertain potentials for profit. Manufacturers will be less likely to invest in the health care technological needs of the less visible, less articulate, and underprivileged groups—the handicapped, the indigent, and the elderly—since support for these technological innovations will be uncertain and slow in coming from public sources. Risks of suppressed or aborted medical innovation due to reimbursement constraints may also be the most damaging effect of cost-containment on the future quality of health care.

Public resources allotted for health care needs have been increasingly perceived to be limited, leading to the belief that decisions to ration access to medical treatment are inevitable (Evans, 1983; Schwartz, 1987). However, rationing is not a concept that is totally foreign to the American system of health care (Mechanic, 1985). Scarce goods and services have always had to be apportioned among needy individuals, and not infrequently, the less affluent have been denied access to expensive technologies. Also, third-party payment mechanisms act as implicit rationing devices, either by imposing coinsurance and deductible payments on patients or by specifying strict criteria governing the context, quantity, setting, and range of reimbursable services.

The cost-containment imperative has led to efforts to limit the growth of the U.S. health care system. For example, the assignment of DRG weights promotes a system of resource allocation per treatment category (Veatch, 1986). In a hospital or other provider institution, resources must be distributed among healthier and sicker patients within a DRG or shifted between profitable and unprofitable DRGs. This leaves institutions, health care professionals, and, to a lesser extent, patients to determine the distribution of health care opportunities and the equity of such trade-offs. This is even more apparent in the capitated practice approach of health maintenance organizations in which the individual is charged on a fixed, periodic prepayment basis regardless of the services he or she has received.

Schwartz (1987) has recently suggested that current cost-control strategies will provide only temporary relief from expansionary health care costs unless future development of new medical technologies is limited and further rationing of services is imposed. The American public, however, has repeatedly demonstrated its great appetite and expectation for increased medical care (Somers, 1986), the importance it places on access to services for the needy (Navarro, 1982), and its unstinting support for biomedical research (Blendon and Altman, 1984). It is hardly conceivable that the American public will be convinced that rationing services of proven benefit or curbing innovation of promising technical advances are in the patient's or even society's best interests. Further, there is no guarantee that the savings that may be realized by rationing health care services will be used more justly or wisely elsewhere (Daniels, 1986). For example, the savings may accrue as profits to entrepreneurs or corporations. Indeed, the design of explicit rationing criteria other than those primarily dealing with issues of quality of care could erode public trust in policymaking and the government (Mechanic, 1985).

This raises the question: "Who should have access to the new medical technologies and why?" (Capron, 1984). There exists a widely acknowledged ethical obligation to provide access to an adequate level of health care for all members of our society (President's Commission for the Study of Ethical Problems in Medicine and Biomedical and Behavioral Research, 1983). To meet this obligation, there needs to be a broad-based decision-making process to judge if the opportunities that are expected to derive from a new technology warrant its inclusion into a "package of benefits" guaranteed to provide an adequate level of health care. Such an assessment should be performed in a timely fashion in order to anticipate future financial requirements, to meet priority health needs, and to establish a rational basis for applying a particular technology efficiently as well as equitably.

An example which illustrates some of these problems is heart transplantation. Medicare issued coverage criteria for heart transplantation in November 1986, long after the procedure was perceived as beneficial and had diffused into accepted clinical practice. It is not inconceivable that the artificial heart and ventricular assist devices may also follow the same path, with failure to deal with their ethical and economic consequences until the technologies are fairly well established and perceived as desirable from the perspectives of physicians as well as the public (Capron, 1984). Unfortunately, although the government is committing a share of its biomedical research funds to the development of these devices, it is also—as regulator and third-party payer—implicitly disavowing responsibility to fund assessments of these new medical devices.

REFORM PROPOSALS

Technology Assessment

Conflicts between cost-containment, access to care, and continued technological progress may never be resolved to the satisfaction of all interested parties. However, attention to improving the timeliness and accountability of coverage payment decision processes will help to make these conflicts less problematic for the health care practitioners and patients who must abide by the decisions. The reimbursement structure does not merely embody a set of prices and allowable charges, but also reflects judgments about relative values and priorities placed on health care services. The challenge is to delineate, with wisdom for the individual and for society, the balance between new health care opportunities and problems created by the introduction and broad application of expensive new medical technologies.

Technology assessment can serve as a tool for reviewing the clinical, social, and economic consequences of a technology and can provide a basis for making policy decisions about resource values. Socially and fiscally responsible coverage and reimbursement policies can work together with technology assessment, both fostering effective and efficient medical care. The primary value of technology assessment for coverage decision making lies in determining the safety and efficacy of medical technologies and discriminating between appropriate and inappropriate indications for use. The reimbursement mechanism can, in turn, generate data needed for technology assessments and serve to implement the conclusions of these assessments.

Technology assessment for coverage decision-making purposes will demand greater analytic resources and augmented data bases than are now available. In making assessments, policymakers and third-party payers should consider issues such as relative efficacy of a new medical technology in comparison with competing technologies; cost-effectiveness; impact on quality of life; rehabilitative potential; the relationship between productivity measures and patient outcomes; and other ethical, legal, and societal concerns.

Beyond coverage decision making, government policy and decisionmakers will have greater concern with the nationwide implications of major new technologies, particularly if—or when—the country institutes some form of a national health program. At present, there is no agency or group in the public or private sector with a mandate to conduct or sponsor such studies, including studies on the potential benefits or hazards of major technologies and their economic and resource costs for the nation. There is no available mechanism through which the nation can deal with the array of issues raised by major technologies, new or existing. Such assessments will require broader input, multidisciplinary expertise, and investment in sophisticated data collection and analysis methods. Certainly the need is pressing, and a possible mechanism for facilitating these assessments may be available in the Council on Health Care Technologies of the Institute of Medicine. Whether the council will move in that direction, or whether a new entity will need to be established, remains to be seen.

One of the most important research areas in technology assessment is the comparison of competing technologies, particularly to determine appropriate clinical indications for use of diagnostic devices (Petitti, 1986). These comparisons can be laborious and difficult, demanding large study populations and complex methodologies. One option would be to provide research support for comparative studies from federal health care delivery dollars. The results of such studies would be of direct value in improving the efficiency of the delivery system and could also lead to more informed and prompt payment decisions. Another, but probably less feasible, approach would be to include preliminary comparative safety data and perhaps even some preliminary cost and efficacy data in the device manufacturer's premarket approval submission to the Food and Drug Administration (FDA) (ECRI, 1986). Although this would add to manufacturers' costs—already considered unduly high—such information could be used as a marketing tool and the costs could be spread over future device sales (ECRI, 1986).

Priority List of Candidate Topics for Assessment and Policy Actions

An important step in improving coverage decision making in Medicare would be to systematically identify priorities among candidate technologies. At present, this is performed on a loosely structured basis, generated in large part by requests from intermediaries and local carriers. Reliance on this method can lead to delays in identifying important coverage concerns and wasting limited resources on nonmeritorious issues. Instead, the coverage process should anticipate issues surrounding new technologies and new applications of existing technologies.

A number of criteria could be adopted to screen new technologies and to order priorities for assessment purposes. These criteria might include medical significance; potential benefit and clinical utility; proportion of beneficiaries affected; spin-off effects; ease of diffusion; economic incentives; impact on the health care delivery system; and important legal, ethical, and social considerations (National Center for Health Care Technology, 1980; Perry, 1982; Roe et al., 1986).

Candidates for assessment could be compiled from a number of sources such as the FDA, the National Institutes of Health, the Public Health Service, the National Center for Health Services Research and Technology Assessment, and the Council on Health Care Technology of the Institute of Medicine. Other professional groups knowledgeable about changes in medical practice could provide expertise and input. These include medical specialty associations, health industry manufacturers' organizations, utilization review groups, and peer review organizations (Roe et al., 1986).

It should be emphasized that the candidate technologies for assessment discussed in this section are not the emerging technologies. Even the identification—let alone the assessment—of such technologies has aroused serious concern from device manufacturers that premature assessment of emerging medical technologies would stifle innovation (Perry, 1982).

Interim Coverage Policy

A decision by the federal government and other third-party payers to cover a particular medical technology need not be all or nothing as it is now. The current situation sometimes fosters enthusiastic adoption of technologies because of overestimation of the number of potential beneficiaries. It also sometimes rewards extravagant application of technology even when marginal cost outweighs marginal benefit. Alternatively, criteria could be more rigorously constructed to define specific indications, circumstances, and qualifications for use. Third-party payers could coordinate efforts with medical specialty societies to encourage the requisite standards for physician training and experience with new procedures and medical device applications. Quality standards for resources, personnel, and participating medical centers could be developed for major, highly specified technologies. Such activities are already under way to a limited extent.

Many procedures can be performed on an outpatient basis safely and less expensively than when provided in a hospital setting. Coverage could be specified to restrict care to the appropriate setting (Greenberg and Derzon, 1981). Regionalization of technologies and procedures requiring highly developed skills and specialized facilities could also be encouraged by third-party payment policies (Perry, 1984). Thus, in coordination with existing local health planning agencies, regional hospital councils, area provider groups, and third-party payers could help discourage duplication of health care services.

Precedents for promoting regionalization of complex medical skills and facilities have been set in both the public and private insurance sectors. In 1982, Blue Shield of California decided to provide coverage for percutaneous transluminal coronary angioplasty only if the physicians were qualified according to criteria set by the National Heart, Lung, and Blood Institute. Medicare has limited payment to specified providers for some procedures, such as therapeutic apheresis, although this has been unusual (Office of Technology Assessment, 1984). In late 1986, Medicare announced that heart transplants would be reimbursed if the transplant centers met certain qualifying criteria. In view of the recent demise of the federal health planning program, third-party payers could play a major role in promoting appropriate regionalization of health care services, thus conserving scarce and expensive resources.

A reform measure recommended by the National Center for Health Care Technology and endorsed by the Office of Technology Assessment would establish interim coverage policies (Office of Technology Assessment, 1984; Towery and Perry, 1981). This could be invoked for expensive, FDA-approved major medical technologies as they enter into the practice setting. Diffusion of the technologies would be limited to selected sites; use would follow predetermined protocols; and reimbursement would be contingent upon collecting early data on safety, effectiveness, relative efficacy, patient outcome, and cost-effectiveness. Such data would provide valuable information on the use of the technology in different clinical settings, information that is not normally collected systematically or in a coordinated fashion.

It is generally the exception, rather than the rule, for a new technology to diffuse in an orderly fashion following the completion of controlled clinical trials, a determination of relative worth, and agreement on appropriate indications for use. An important current example is the MRI. Opinions may differ about the appropriate rate of diffusion of MRI, but there is little disagreement that studies of its clinical value have not proceeded in a rational manner. Acquisition has largely been based on considerations other than clinical benefit (Hillman and Schwartz, 1986).

It may be difficult to prevent premature diffusion of new medical devices because the collection and reporting of data from health care delivery systems is greatly deficient. A new technology may not be identified on insurance claims or may be hidden within an existing procedure, thus forfeiting the opportunity to study its costs and outcomes (Bunker et al., 1982). An interim coverage policy not only provides a sounder basis for more permanent coverage decisions but also adds coherence to the development and evaluation of technologies entering the health care delivery system. ProPAC also has considered developing device-specific temporary DRGs for new medical technologies (Technology Reimbursement Reports, 1986). This approach would monitor practice patterns and price changes for new technologies prior to a permanent DRG assignment. Criteria for a permanent assignment would relate to the costs of the new technology and other technologies within the DRG, the differences in clinical utility and resource use related to the new technology, and evidence of adverse impacts on access.

Senators David Durenburger (R, Minn.) and Lloyd Bentsen (D, Tex.) introduced a bill (S. 2474) in the 1986 legislative session and again in the 1987 session (S. 897) that would target funds for temporary Medicare coverage of FDA-approved technologies. Medicare would pay 60 percent of the added costs for the approved technology for those cases that cost more than 110 percent of the DRG rate. The temporary coverage would be in effect for a trial period of 2 years, during which data concerning effectiveness and costs of the new technology would be submitted to help formulate a permanent coverage decision.

However, these policy proposals do not set priorities among new technologies, as would a selective interim coverage policy. This proposal would also necessitate estimating costs of a new technology, which would be a complicated task (Garrison and Wilensky, 1986). And although interim coverage provides support at a critical juncture between marketing and reimbursement, the level of coverage may still be insufficient for some providers and patients.

Hospital claim forms for reimbursement appear to be inefficient sources of data on new devices and their complications and outcomes. Confusion and misunderstandings over which code to use can lead to inconsistencies in reporting the use of new medical devices. The classification system used in Medicare's PPS is the International Classification of Diseases, Ninth Revision, Clinical Modification (ICD–9-CM). A formal mechanism for coding recommendations, formulating new procedural codes, and providing coordination between HCFA and the National Center of Health Statistics has recently been established (Office of Technology Assessment, 1985b). But no current codes describe misapplication, malfunction, failure, or other device-related complications or distinguish between the many device models. Some of these changes are proposed for the 10th revision of the ICD-CM (Thacker and Berkelman, 1986).

A recent survey noted that hospitals' device-related problems were not reported to outside organizations, such as the FDA or medical device manufacturers, 49 percent of the time (General Accounting

Office, 1986). Claims data and postmarketing surveillance networks are potentially valuable sources for information on device practice patterns and should be made more useful.

Periodic Payment Adjustments

A reimbursement structure should be responsive to and provide appropriate incentives for beneficial technological change. Medical progress does not always advance in a step-by-step, straightforward fashion. Instead, it may draw upon a mix of contributions from a broad array of sciences and fortuitous discoveries (Moloney and Rogers, 1979). A reimbursement structure cannot feasibly acknowledge each minor step in the evolution of a technology's development and refinement, nor should it. However, recognition of the cumulative iterative process and interim products of the learning and development phases of a technology (Feeny, 1985) could help maintain the sensitivity of payment rates to ongoing practice patterns.

In a fixed-rate reimbursement system, periodic adjustments are needed in order to maintain the correlation between payments and the cost of efficient care (Office of Technology Assessment, 1985b). If a cost-saving technology is introduced, or if the cost of a technology decreased after the initial phases of development, the per-case payment should reflect this decrease. Likewise, the use of costly innovations that prove to be advantageous for diagnostic efficiency or treatment should elicit an upward adjustment in payments. Such an evolutionary process would more evenhandedly encourage the diffusion of both cost-saving and cost-increasing, but beneficial, technologies.

Charges for the application of expensive devices should be better defined in order to verify the calculation of DRG weights. In some DRGs, the inclusion of costly device-related cases with cases where such devices are not used may suggest that patient characteristics are distinct and may warrant reclassification in order to maintain DRG homogeneity (Prospective Payment Assessment Commission, 1986c). Two or more types of a medical device can be used for patients within the same diagnosis or treatment group, but may vary significantly in resource costs. For example, four DRG categories describe patient groups requiring pacemaker implantation. There are also four major device types, each with a different cost. This distinction is not recognized in the existing DRG rate structure (Altman, 1985). ProPAC has recommended that the grouping of pacemaker implantations be reclassified in order to correlate resource use with payment rates more effectively (Prospective Payment Assessment Commission, 1986b), but this recommendation was rejected by HCFA.

Greater Public Input into Coverage Decision Making

Promulgating clearly defined rules and criteria governing coverage and payment policy decisions would improve the accountability and reliability of such decisions (Roe et al., 1986). Until recently, HCFA has not made public its rules regarding national coverage decisions, perhaps because they were not explicit. The absence of a clear understanding of this process bars effective public participation and appeal and may lead to geographical variations in coverage policy. If the steps involved in appealing for additional reimbursement for a new technology or if the rationale for denial of coverage are unknown, then manufacturers, physicians, and patients are unable to challenge such decisions on a rational basis.

Coverage decision-making processes should also permit greater public participation by hospital providers and patients (Roe et al., 1986). Presently, there is no opportunity for public review of the reports of the Office of Health Technology Assessment before the policy determinations are made by HCFA. Disclosure of coverage policy decisions would encourage responses and recommendations from experts and interested groups. In turn, these groups could submit relevant economic or clinical data related to the coverage decision.

Impartial advisory boards composed of clinicians, health professionals, policy analysts, economists, and others could fulfill an important function in ensuring that the coverage process responds to the needs of the health care community. Congress established an independent body, ProPAC, to help provide fairness and objectivity in setting hospital rates (Verville, 1985). However, a number of DRG adjustments proposed by ProPAC in response to changing medical practices were rejected by HCFA. In some cases, Congress itself has enacted adjustments to hospital payments (Prospective Payment Assessment Commission, 1986d). ProPAC's deliberations and recommendations should be afforded greater weight, and there should be mechanisms to provide review and a recourse to appeal HCFA's reimbursement decisions (ECRI, 1986).

Identification of Outmoded, Ineffective, and Overutilized Existing Technologies

There are few data on the continued use of technologies that are ineffective or have been superseded by superior technologies; indiscriminate application of old or existing technologies is fairly common. Present reimbursement procedures on the whole do not discourage such practices, and in fact, PPS tends to make them even less visible.

Identification and elimination of outdated technologies has, on the whole, been neglected, although a great deal has been said and written about the subject.

New evidence may warrant a reassessment of an already covered service or a technology that has been denied coverage. Such evidence may include advances in the state of the art, the introduction of alternative techniques, emerging safety concerns, new evidence about the effectiveness of a procedure or device, or refinement of clinical applications. Additional criteria for selecting old technologies for review could include the magnitude of the economic impact of competing technologies—including both prevalence of practice and cost per unit, potential for misuse, feasibility of an assessment, or evidence of cost-ineffectiveness of an outdated device or procedure (National Center for Health Care Technology, 1980). Based on periodic review, coverage for these technologies could be eliminated, redefined, or limited.

CONCLUSION

In this era of cost-containment, there is increasing discussion of the issues surrounding quality of care; thus far, there has been relatively little action. No longer are improvements in health or expansions in access to care heralded as a mark of success. Instead, total savings now serve as the yardstick of achievement for health benefits programs (Eisenberg, 1984). As third-party payers, self-insurers, and other parties increasingly intervene to mandate service utilization patterns and clinical practices, they should also accept partial responsibility for the consequent health outcomes.

A comprehensive effort should be undertaken to monitor the impact of alternative payment systems. Technological change, access, and quality of care should all be evaluated.

These studies should also seek to identify significant "spillover" effects into other components of the health care delivery system. If an economically oriented reimbursement system inadvertently creates hardship for hospitals providing public services, if patients are unable to gain access to medical care for financial reasons, or if there is a redistribution of the gains of technological change from the less wealthy to the more wealthy, then the social costs of such programs are too high.

Research of this type needs to be conducted before a new reimbursement program is established. Relatively little was known about the long-term impact of the PPS on both costs and quality of care prior to its institution nationally. Any thought of changing to another mode of reimbursement, such as capitation, should be accompanied by foresight, planning, and testing.

Ultimately, cost-containment strategies must redirect funds away from unnecessary and ineffective care and toward effective medical care (Angell, 1985). The primary obstacle to distinguishing effective medical care from care of little or unproven value is lack of knowledge and data on new and existing technologies (Jennett, 1984). Public sector investments in primary data collection have decreased at the same time that the needs to improve and refine coverage policy—and the subsequent need for more and better data—have accelerated.

The Institute of Medicine has recommended that "payment for medical technology assessment should be made through the system that pays for medical care." Such funds could be raised either by "a set-aside percentage of the health care dollar" (Institute of Medicine, 1985), as has been proposed previously, or by a per capita levy on insurers (Bunker et al., 1982; Relman, 1982). As Arnold Relman, the editor of the *New England Journal of Medicine*, notes, "It is the cost of this ignorance, not of medical progress, that has now become too steep for us to bear. The cost culprit is not technology per se, but only technology that is ineffective, superfluous or unsafe" (Relman, 1982).

It is time for the government, insurers, manufacturers, and providers to embrace common objectives and to acknowledge and fully support the crucial role of medical technology assessment in the enhancement of the quality of health care and the discriminate and equitable use of scarce resources. To ignore this need through preoccupation with management by numbers or reliance on cost-competitive choices would be seriously shortsighted and an injustice to our society.

REFERENCES

Altman, S. H. 1985. Will the Medicare Prospective Payment System succeed? Technical adjustments can make the difference. Arthur Weissman Memorial Lecture, University of California, Berkeley, School of Public Health.

Anderson, G., and E. Steinberg. 1984. To buy or not to buy: Technology acquisition under prospective payment. New England Journal of Medicine 311:182–185.

Angell, M. 1985. Cost containment and the physician. Journal of the American Medical Association 254:1203–1207.

Bessey, E. C. 1986. Don't let cost containment stifle technological innovation. Medical Marketing and Media 21:8–10, 14–16.

Blendon, R. J., and D. E. Altman. 1984. Public attitudes about health care costs: A lesson in national schizophrenia. New England Journal of Medicine 311:613–616.

Bunker, J. P., and R. W. Schaffarzick. 1986. Reimbursement incentives for hospital care. Annual Review of Public Health 7:391–409.

Bunker, J. P., J. Fowles, and R. W. Schaffarzick. 1982. Evaluation of medical technology strategies: Proposal for an Institute for Health Care Evaluation. New England Journal of Medicine 306:620–624, 687–692.

Capron, A. M. 1984. An ethical obligation to ensure access to new medical technologies? Journal of Health Care Technology 1:103–120.

Daniels, N. 1986. Why saying no to patients in the United States is so hard: Cost containment, justice and provider autonomy. New England Journal of Medicine 314:1380–1383.

Detsky, A. S. 1987. Decision analysis: What's the prognosis? Annals of Internal Medicine 106:321–322.

ECRI. 1986. Medicare payment for new technologies—Can the process be improved despite conflicting goals? Journal of Health Care Technology 3:13–32.

Eisenberg, L. 1984. Rudolf Ludwig Karl Virchow, where are you now that we need you? American Journal of Medicine 77:524–532.

Evans, R. W. 1983. Health care technology and the inevitability of resource allocation and rationing decisions. Journal of the American Medical Association 249:2047–2053, 2209–2219.

Feeny, D. 1986. Neglected issues in the diffusion of health care technologies: The role of skills and learning. International Journal of Technology Assessment 1:681–692.

Finkelstein, S. N., K. A. Isaacson, and J. J. Frishkopf. 1984. The process of evaluating medical technologies for third-party coverage. Journal of Health Care Technology 1:89–102.

Fruen, M. A., and H. A. DiPrete. 1986. Health Care in the Future. Boston, Mass.: John Hancock Mutual Life Insurance Company.

Garrison, L. P., and G. R. Wilensky. 1986. Cost containment and incentives for technology. Health Affairs 5:46–58.

General Accounting Office. 1985. Information Requirements for Evaluating the Impacts of Medicare Prospective Payment on Post-Hospital Long-Term Care Services: Preliminary Report. GAO/PEMD–85–8. Washington, D.C.: U.S. Government Printing Office.

General Accounting Office. 1986. Medical Devices: Early Warning of Problems Is Hampered by Severe Underreporting. GAO/PEMP–87–1. Washington, D.C.: U.S. Government Printing Office.

Ginzberg, E. 1984. The monetarization of medical care. New England Journal of Medicine 310:1162–1165.

Greenberg, B., and R. A. Derzon. 1981. Determining health insurance coverage of technology: Problems and options. Medical Care 19:967–978.

Hillman, A. 1986. Government health policy and the diffusion of new medical devices. Health Services Research 21:680–711.

Hillman, A. S., and J. S. Schwartz. 1986. The diffusion of MRI: Patterns of siting and ownership in an era of changing incentives. American Journal of Radiology 146:963–969.

Iglehart, J. K. 1986. Health policy report: Early experience with prospective payment of hospitals. New England Journal of Medicine 314:1460–1464.

Institute of Medicine. 1985. Assessing Medical Technologies. Washington, D.C.: National Academy Press.

Institute of Medicine. 1986. For-Profit Enterprise in Medicine. Washington, D.C.: National Academy Press.

Jennett, B. 1984. High-technology medicine: Benefits and burdens. London: The Nuffield Provincial Hospital Trusts.

Mechanic, D. 1985. Cost containment and the quality of medical care: Rationing strategies in an era of constrained resources. Milbank Memorial Fund Quarterly/ Health and Society 63:453–475.

Merrill, J. C., and R. J. Wasserman. 1985. Growth in national expenditures: Additional analyses. Health Affairs 4:91–97.

Moloney, T. W., and D. E. Rogers. 1979. Medical technology—A different view of the contentious debate over costs. New England Journal of Medicine 301:1413–1419.

Myers, L. P., and S. A. Schroeder. 1981. Physician use of services for the hospitalized patient: A review, with implications for cost containment. Milbank Memorial Fund Quarterly/Health and Society 59:481–507.

National Center for Health Care Technology. 1980. Procedures, Priorities and Policy for the Assessment of Health Care Technology. Washington, D.C.: U.S. Government Printing Office.

Navarro, V. 1982. Sounding boards: Where is the popular mandate? New England Journal of Medicine 307:1516–1518.

Office of Technology Assessment. 1984. Medical Technology and the Costs of the Medicare Program. OTA-H–227. Washington, D.C.: U.S. Government Printing Office.

Office of Technology Assessment. 1985a. Technology and Aging in America. OTA-BA– 264. Washington, D.C.: U.S. Government Printing Office.

Office of Technology Assessment. 1985b. Medicare's PPS—Strategies for Evaluating Costs, Quality and Medical Technology. OTA-H–262. Washington, D.C.: U.S. Government Printing Office.

Perry, S. 1982. The brief life of the National Center for Health Care Technology. New England Journal of Medicine 307:1095–1100.

Perry, S. 1984. Rational and irrational diffusion of new technologies. Journal of Health Care Technology 1:73–88.

Petitti, D. B. 1986. Competing technologies: Implications for the costs and complexity of medical care. New England Journal of Medicine 315:1480–1483.

President's Commission for the Study of Ethical Problems in Medicine and Biomedical and Behavioral Research. 1983. Securing Access to Health Care: The Ethical Implications of Differences in the Availability of Health Services, Volume 1: Report. Washington, D.C.: U.S. Government Printing Office.

Prospective Payment Assessment Commission. 1985. Report and Recommendations to the Secretary, U.S. Department of Health and Human Services, April 1, 1985. Washington, D.C.: Prospective Payment Assessment Commission.

Prospective Payment Assessment Commission. 1986b. Report and Recommendations to the Secretary, U.S. Department of Health and Human Services. Washington, D.C.: Prospective Payment Assessment Commission.

Prospective Payment Assessment Commission. 1986c. Report and Recommendations with Technical Appendixes to the Secretary, U.S. Department of Health and Human Services. Washington, D.C.: Prospective Payment Assessment Commission.

Prospective Payment Assessment Commission. 1986d. 1987 Adjustments to the Medicare Prospective Payment System: Report to the Congress. Washington, D.C.: Prospective Payment Assessment Commission.

Prospective Payment Assessment Commission. 1987. Medicare Prospective Payment and the American Health Care System: Report to the Congress. Washington, D.C.: Prospective Payment Assessment Commission.

Reiser, S. J. 1978. Medicine and the Reign of Technology. Cambridge, England: Cambridge University Press.

Relman, A. S. 1982. An institute for health care evaluation. New England Journal of Medicine 306:669–670.

Relman, A. S. 1985. Antitrust law and the physician entrepreneur. New England Journal of Medicine 313:884–885.

Roe, W., M. Anderson, J. Gong, and M. Strauss. 1986. A forward plan for Medicare coverage and technology assessment. Prepared for the Assistant Secretary of Planning and Evaluation, U.S. Department of Health and Human Services. Washington, D.C.: Lewin and Associates.

Roe, W. I. 1985. Medical technology under PPS: An uncertain future. Hospitals 59:88–92.

Ruby, G., H. D. Banta, and A. K. Burns. 1985. Medicare coverage, Medicare costs and medical technology. Journal of Health Politics, Policy and Law 10:141–155.

Schwartz, W. B. 1987. The inevitable failure of current cost-containment strategies. Why they can provide only temporary relief. Journal of the American Medical Association 257:220–224.

Somers, A. R. 1986. The changing demand for health services: A historical perspective and some thoughts for the future. Inquiry 23:395–402.

Steinberg, E. P., J. E. Sisk, and K. E. Locke. 1985. X-ray CT and magnetic resonance imagers: Diffusion patterns and policy issues. New England Journal of Medicine 313:859–864.

Technology Reimbursement Reports. 1986. Temporary "Device-Specific" DRGs should be used for some new technologies, ProPAC recommends. Technology Reimbursement Reports 2:2.

Thacker, S. B., and R. L. Berkelman. 1986. Surveillance of Medical Technologies. Journal of Public Health Policy 7:363–377.

Towery, O. B., and S. Perry. 1981. The scientific basis for coverage decisions by third-party payers. Journal of the American Medical Association 245:59–61.

Veatch, R. M. 1986. DRGs and the ethical reallocation of resources. Hastings Center Report 16:32–40.

Verville, R. E. 1985. Medicare rate setting and its problems: A fixed price per bundled product. Journal of Legal Medicine 6:85–106.

White, J. K. 1985. Data watch: Health care innovation in an era of cost containment. Health Affairs 4:105–118.

Part 3
How Trends
Will Interact

How Trends Will Interact:
The Perspective of the Hospital

JOHN H. MOXLEY III AND PENELOPE C. ROEDER

When the 62-year old patient entered [the medical center] last spring, he never expected to walk out of the . . . hospital the next day. After two unsuccessful attempts at surgical removal of the fat deposits clogging an artery in his left leg, some doctors concluded that an amputation was the only way to stop the severe pain. But a team of surgeons . . . decided to make one last try with a risky and highly experimental technique that had never been used on a human. The team snaked an optical fiber into the clogged blood vessel and then shot laser light through it, vaporizing the blockage. Less than 24 hours later, the patient went home. His only medication: aspirin.

This story is not science fiction or creative speculation; it is an item reported in the October 17, 1983, issue of *Business Week*.

The fact is, most of us have become somewhat jaded because the things that we think of as advanced technology are already so pervasive in the medicine of the late 1980s. As a result, we often do not know whether to count our blessings or bemoan our fate as we consider the obstacles to the further progress of technologies.

Neither the complexities of, nor the questions surrounding, development of medical technologies are new areas of concern. In 1968 members of the President's Science Advisory Committee (PSAC) considered many of these issues in regard to funding of the National Institutes of Health (NIH). In *The Youngest Science*, Lewis Thomas describes PSAC's findings:

We recognized three levels of medical technology: (1) genuine high technology, exemplified by Salk and Sabin poliomyelitis vaccines, which simply eliminated a major disease at very low cost by providing protection against the three strains of virus known to exist; (2) "halfway" technology, applied to the management of disease when the underlying mechanism is not understood and when medicine is obliged to do whatever it can to shore up and postpone incapacitation and death, at whatever cost, usually very high cost indeed, illustrated by open-heart surgery, coronary artery by-pass, and the replacement of damaged organs by transplanting new ones (at extremely high cost); and (3) nontechnology, the kind of things doctors do when there is nothing at all to be done, as in the care of patients with advanced cancer and senile dementia. *We suggested that the rising cost of health care was resulting from efforts to treat diseases of the halfway or nontechnology class, and recommended that more basic research on these ailments be sponsored by NIH* (emphasis added) (Thomas, 1983, pp. 264–265).

There is, however, a significant question that was not addressed by the PSAC—not the question of whether new technologies can or *should* be used, but whether they *will* be used. This question was of little interest in 1968, when it was assumed that all technology would be used. Nearly 20 years later, in an environment of constrained resources, the question of what will actually happen at the level of the provider/patient interface has become a critical issue.

We examine this critical issue primarily from the perspective of hospitals where administrators make decisions daily that may affect the availability and use of new technologies. We also examine briefly the participation of payers through appropriateness review, as well as some of the societal issues that affect providers, payers, and patients.

Before discussing the specific issues, it is important to set the stage by looking briefly at the practice of medicine and its relation to hospitals and technology development.

Since World War II there have been at least four significant changes in the health care environment. These include increased funding for biomedical research, dramatic growth in the availability of health insurance, rapid rises in the numbers and types of medical specialists and subspecialists, and expanding use of medical technologies.

The relationship between the financing changes and the changes in medical practice patterns can be briefly summarized in a single sentence: With few limits on the availability of funds, medical practices were often based on the belief that more care was better care.

The relationship between the rise of specialty medicine and the spread of technology is no less important. As new technologies have become available, new groups of physicians have become specialized in their use. For example, cardiology now encompasses invasive and noninvasive cardiologists. Lithotripsy has given birth to a whole new group of urologists, as in vitro fertilization has to obstetricians/gynecologists. With recent developments in magnetic resonance imaging (MRI), it would not be surprising to see the growth of MRI subspecialists in a host of current specialists. From a hospital's perspective, each of these technological developments has given rise to a special interest group that can dramatically affect not only the institution's governance but also its capital and operating decisions.

After more than a generation of medical practice dominated by nearly open-ended financing and growth in medical specialties and widely disseminated, complex technologies, we still find ourselves in a world in which most of our medical resources are devoted to the kind of acute-care medicine Dr. Thomas (1983) and his colleagues labeled "halfway technologies."

Although we may be closer to discovering the "high technologies," there has not yet been quite enough time. We still need more research to transform our recent progress in genetic engineering into actual cures of Alzheimer's disease or multiple sclerosis; we still need more research to develop the neural prostheses that can change the lives of trauma victims and that can enable the blind to see and the deaf to hear.

THE PERSPECTIVE OF HEALTH CARE PAYERS

Today we have entered a new world—a world in which the costs of health care are increasingly monitored by payers from both the public and private sectors. Although we can argue that high technologies would reduce society's total health care bill over the long term, today's payers have found that they can save far more by looking first at the simple issues of how care is delivered for some very common occurrences such as back pain, normal obstetrical deliveries, and children's sore throats. While these payers clearly hope to reduce the costs of treating all illness—including the more complex cases of cancer and heart disease—they hope to do so by *effecting fundamental changes in the current medical care system.*

Let us look at the changes sought by payers and think about the impact they will have on the adoption of new medical technologies.

The most obvious fact about the new health care environment is the alphabet soup of new delivery networks. Whether these groups are called health maintenance organizations (HMOs), preferred provider organizations (PPOs), or anything else, they tend to have a number of features which can have an impact on the technology adoption process. Perhaps most important, most have a single agent—an insurance company, the employer group itself, or some other intermediary—that administers payment for all services delivered to plan members. This is not a simple check-writing function; it is a true oversight function.

While reviewers may check invoices submitted by providers for billing errors and price levels, their *primary* function is to *review the appropriateness of the care delivered.* However, many of these reviewers base their assessments of appropriateness more on financial averages than on clinical considerations. There is, therefore, an increasing tendency to review claims on the basis of costs per case rather than on the needs of a particular patient.

THE PERSPECTIVE OF THE HOSPITAL

Whether it is based on clinical expertise or not, this kind of appropriateness review has become part of the clinical decision-making process. It has also put the hospital in the middle of the clinical decision-making process by forcing it to act as the payer's local policeman. If the hospital does not accept this role, it is often forced to forgo payment for services and to withstand some financial loss.

Appropriateness review has also forced some dramatic shifts in the ways in which hospitals adopt new technologies. A brief review of those shifts will help illuminate their possible long-term impact on the development and use of new medical technologies.

All providers—be they not-for-profit or investor-owned institutions, solo physicians, or members of group practices—are able to continue delivering medical care only if they can meet the costs of doing business. That is, all of them must generate an economic profit, whatever name they choose to apply to it.

In the cost-based payment environment that existed until a few years ago, virtually all services delivered were profitable. That is no longer the case. In 1983 the federal government introduced prospective pricing by diagnostic-related groups (DRGs). Increasingly, private payers are also adopting the prospective pricing principle. When prices are set prospectively, profit is earned only when the costs of producing a product are less than the prices paid for the product.

If this point seems trivial, that is only because it reflects the basic economics under which most American industries have operated for decades. For the health care world steeped in cost-based reimbursement, it is, however, an unfamiliar perspective. Prospective pricing has forced providers to revise the way they think about such things as capital investments, operating expenses, and market share.

Despite the fact that hospitals' expenses have not been included under DRGs, there was a decrease in those expenses in 1984 and 1985. In 1986 capital expenditures rose in what many believe was the anticipation that they would soon be integrated into the DRG system. There are now clear indications that many hospitals are considering or have implemented reductions in capital expenditures. In December 1986, for example, Thomas Frist, the chief executive officer of Hospital Corporation of America, announced that capital spending had been cut from $1.4 billion in 1985 to about $700 million in 1986 (McGraw-Hill's Health Business, 1987). Certainly, some of the industry-wide reduction in capital expenditures has been in response to a generally tighter economic environment. However, in some hospitals it also reflects a completely new approach to capital budgeting.

Rigorous economic analysis has not always been part of most hospitals' decision-making process. Indeed, most hospital analysts have concentrated on developing their reimbursement savvy, and few have had the traditional capital budgeting skills found in other industries.

It used to be that hospitals made purchasing decisions based entirely on physician demand, and that physicians demanded whatever tools or procedures they were comfortable with—often without regard to the cost. Hospital boards or managements might have decided against a project, but that was more often for reasons of timing or overall desirability than it was for economic reasons.

The results of decision making based on physician demand are now apparent throughout the country. For example, it is not uncommon to see cardiac catheterization laboratories in small rural or semirural hospitals with a single cardiologist and one trained technician. It is difficult to believe that the incremental patient load brought to most rural hospitals by such a service is likely to justify the cost of a trained technician and the capital investment required to run the lab. In fact, administrators of some of these hospitals use their small patient loads as justification for cardiac catheterization prices that are higher than those at the large medical center 2 hours away.

Certainly, such an investment would be made on the basis of clinical factors: There is ample evidence that the risk factors for patients in this kind of situation are high (Shortell and LoGerfo, 1981; Showstack et al., 1987). Instead, such investment decisions have been based on the assumption that any additional services—and any additional patients—would be profitable under the payment systems that were in place.

In the current environment, however, even rigorous economic analyses are only marginally useful for hospital managers attempting to make rational capital investment decisions. This point is easily illustrated by a number of examples.

The first involves the coverage of a new technology under the DRG system. DRG no. 108 prescribes the reimbursement rate for cardiothoracic procedures, except valve and coronary bypass, with pump;

it has a weight of 4.7810. When DRGs were originally introduced, this DRG included angioplasty. With that basis of payment, any hospital that handled a reasonable number of patients with obstructed coronary arteries (procedure code 36.0) was likely to invest in angioplasty: It was much less costly to deliver than the alternative procedures covered by the DRG.

Within a short period of time, however, a new procedure code was introduced for angioplasty and the procedure was moved to another DRG (no. 112; vascular procedures except major reconstruction, without pump) with a weighting of 2.2239. At an average blended DRG rate of $3,000, this change reduced payment for each angioplasty by more than $7,600. At the very least, the projected return from the investment in angioplasty was considerably diminished.

A second example involves another new technology—this time a very expensive piece of equipment: the lithotriptor, which provides noninvasive treatment of the common kidney stone. From a clinical perspective, a lithotriptor appears to be a desirable investment. From an economic perspective, it would also appear to be reasonable at first glance, since noninvasive procedures generally reduce hospitalization time—and costs—for patients. However, that rationale does not take into account the realities of reimbursement: When the Health Care Financing Administration decided to reimburse lithotripsy, they decided to cover it as a medical, not a surgical, procedure. DRG no. 323, medical treatment of a kidney stone, pays only half as much as DRG no. 308, which applies to the surgical treatment of kidney stones. In effect, this means that many hospitals that could serve a sizable patient base with a lithotriptor simply cannot justify the investment on an economic basis.

We emphasize that we are not commenting on the logic or the justness of these reimbursement decisions. Rather, we would argue that such decisions—particularly if made abruptly—make reasonable analysis of capital investments very difficult for the hospital. Faced with such uncertainty, hospitals are apt to adopt progressively more conservative capital investment postures which may well slow the rate of introduction of new and "higher" technology into the health care system.

It is arguable that the current reimbursement policy will force a centralization of lithotriptors in regional referral centers, and that may be a good thing. Nevertheless, it is certainly a different pattern than the one followed by the diffusion of computerized axial tomography (CT scanning). The example of CT scanning is, of course, a telling one: At its introduction in the mid-1970s, the CT scanner was one of the leading drivers of health planning. Many argued that its dissemination would contribute significantly to the rapid escalation of health care costs. In retrospect, we now know that the capabilities of CT scanning and the improved ability to do noninvasive diagnostic work have in fact *reduced* the net cost of treating some diseases—most notably, neurological disease (Altman and Blendon, 1979).

This example illustrates an important point: To the extent that dissemination of technology becomes dependent on prospective financial analyses, we may miss opportunities to reduce the net costs of health care. Among other things, we will remove the opportunity for many creative physicians to develop new and effective applications of these technologies and therapies. On the other hand, if we allow new technologies to be disseminated as before, without careful attention to their cost-effective uses, increases in health care costs may indeed outweigh the benefits of these technologies.

If society is to continue to benefit from the development of new technologies that require significant capital investments, we must have more information than has traditionally been provided by clinical trials. In addition to data about clinical effectiveness, we must know the specific advantages of the new technology—how it will improve the delivery of care and what its rational relationships with other technologies may be. Only if the cost-effective use of new equipment can be demonstrated to both providers and payers will providers be able to count on reimbursement and make the necessary investments to adopt the new technology in this economically driven environment. While these expanded clinical trials will be more expensive, the logical source of payment is the payers that will benefit significantly from the expanded data base and reduced costs of care.

Tests of cost-effectiveness also will be applied to routine clinical activities in hospitals. Consider, for example, intravenous therapy. The protocols for starting intravenous therapy are highly variable throughout the United States. Even within a single system of hospitals, differences in the amount of tape, the kinds and amount of packing, and the types of needles and catheters used can result in variations of 250 percent per insertion in the cost of materials for this simple procedure. Add to this the variability of hospital rules about the frequency of reinserting the intravenous line, and there exists an opportunity for significant unnecessary expenditures (R. M. Schlosser, personal communication).

This example, like those that preceded it, is not raised for the value of its particulars. Instead, all of them are provided as illustrations of a new approach to acquiring and using biotechnical materials. Increasingly, providers will undertake careful analyses of all purchases to ensure that they provide cost-effective care and, hence, are likely to be reimbursed.

However, these examples leave out the important issue of market share and its effect on the adoption of new technologies. Historically, one of the major reasons for hospitals to invest in new technologies was to expand services. In theory, such expansion would attract more patients, thereby increasing the hospital's market share.

In the economically driven environment, growth in market share will continue to provide a strong motivation to adopt new technologies and devices. However, the hospitals' pursuit of market share will focus on technologies that will increase profits. Under cost-plus reimbursement, virtually any technology that physicians used increased profits, even if only a few patients were served. In the current environment of price constraints, however, new technologies must serve enough patients to more than cover the costs of equipment and specially trained personnel.

Even with better understanding of the clinical advantages of new technologies, economic forces are likely to encourage centralization of expensive equipment. This centralization is likely to reduce patients' access to some kinds of health care. Payers' increased participation in individual beneficiaries' care, as well as increases in patients' copayments and deductibles, will accentuate that trend. To the degree that we believe that society is suffering from the overuse of health services, these changes may be beneficial.

Some observers of the health care scene are quite explicit in their beliefs that curbing the development and diffusion of clinically useful technologies may be the only way to achieve long-term control of health care costs. They argue that even low-risk new technologies with low unit costs add to net health care costs because they are used on many more patients. Thus, they argue, we ought to limit the development and use of new technology (Schwartz, 1987).

However, in its extreme, this approach seems to be little different than the traditional rationing approach—except, perhaps, in the sense that we allow ourselves to claim that we have not made prior decisions about which class of patients will be ineligible for which set of benefits. We would argue that there are more productive ways to make policy than by using what might be called "simple default by economics." Indeed, there may be better ways to develop even more cost-effective strategies.

Interestingly, even the most adamant proponents of rationing are beginning to recognize that there may be more productive ways to allocate medical resources than by price manipulations and other simple marketplace strategies. They are beginning to advocate that we learn where sound clinical management can contribute to economic savings.

The need to improve clinical management is being advocated not only by clinicians but also by both public and private sector payers. As reductions in resources available to pay for health care have raised fears of inadequate medical care among health care consumers, some payers have begun to develop more sophisticated ways to monitor the delivery of care (Roeder and Moxley, 1986).

The availability of large computers that can house massive data bases, coupled with the need to balance costs and quality of medical care, has encouraged increasing analysis of clinical records. Many payers, who have records for and are responsible for meeting commitments to patients in a variety of treatment settings, are beginning longitudinal studies. The data in these tracking systems are being analyzed to determine where strong correlations between treatments and outcomes exist. Where negative correlations are found, even low-cost treatments will be proscribed; where there are positive outcomes, higher-cost treatments are likely to become the treatment of choice.

Few payers have yet developed this level of sophistication in their analysis; most are still trying to determine when outpatient treatment is more cost-effective than hospitalization. However, interest in the area has given impetus to the work of C. N. Wennberg at Dartmouth and R. H. Brook and his colleagues at the Rand Corporation. On the basis of his work, Brook advocates careful study of the risks and benefits of technologies in a variety of settings—ranging from academic medical centers with specially trained staff to community hospitals with their medical staffs—as well as the use of formal decision analysis by physicians. Such informed choice, Brook argues, can reduce the growth of health care expenditures sufficiently to permit the continued development and appropriate diffusion of new technologies (Brook and Lohr, 1986).

Until the level of sophistication aimed at by Brook and his colleagues is more widely available, we are likely to see the delivery of some shortsighted, low-cost, but ultimately ineffective, medical care. In such situations, conflicts between cost-conscious payers and clinically oriented providers are inevitable.

One of the primary responsibilities of the scientific community in this transitional period will be to help providers develop the data necessary to measure the effectiveness of care and to make the case for continuing use of appropriate new technologies. Only if we are able to work together in this effort will we be able to avoid the error of applying simple solutions to complex problems by relying solely on market forces to curb the development of technology.

CONCLUSION

In this paper we have examined some of the recent changes in health care financing and the ways that they are affecting the adoption of new technologies. The relevant changes include increasingly restricted financial resources for health care, payers' attempts to effect fundamental changes in medical care, payers' increasing involvement in clinical decision making through the claims review process and consequent pressure on health care institutions to administer financial controls or incur costs themselves, and health care institutions' early efforts to respond to changed conditions by adopting new rules for economic investment decisions. We have also discussed briefly how those new rules could lead to a form of economic rationing of health care services.

We do not believe that this outcome is inevitable. The work of Brook, Wennberg, and the many others who are beginning to respond to Earnest Codman's 1913 call for research on medical outcomes should provide much encouragement to all of us. However, the biomedical community must remain vigilant—and expend the time and energy required to be constructive participants in the policymaking process—if we as a society are to avoid the adoption of the deceptively simple solution of economic rationing.

This is a significant responsibility for the scientific community to accept. However, its participation is essential to the successful resolution of these important issues. To quote again from Lewis Thomas: "It is a gamble to bet on science for moving ahead, but it is, in my view, the only game in town" (Thomas, 1984).

If we are to continue to benefit from the single most important characteristic of twentieth century U.S. medicine—its capacity for scientific improvement and technological adaptation—we must ensure that the public and private sectors understand the importance of, and work together to support, advances in science and technology.

REFERENCES

Altman, S. H., and R. J. Blendon, eds. 1979. Medical Technology: The Culprit Behind Health Care Costs? Publication No. (PHS) 79–3216. Washington, D.C.: U.S. Department of Health, Education, and Welfare.

Brook, R. H., and K. N. Lohr. 1986. Will we need to ration effective health care? Issues in Science and Technology 3(1):68–77.

BusinessWeek. 1983. How laser surgery is moving medicine light years ahead. October 17, 1983.

McGraw-Hill's Health Business. 1987. HCA: Plenty of rigging for the long haul, but smooth sailing—A receding memory. McGraw Hill's Health Business 2(16):1T.

Roeder, P. C., and J. H. Moxley III. 1986. How does the profit motive affect the quality of care? The For-Profit Hospital, Richard F. Southby and Warren Greenberg, eds. Columbus: Battelle Press.

Schwartz, W. B. 1987. The inevitable failure of current cost-containment strategies. Journal of the American Medical Association 257(2):220–224.

Shortell, S. M., and J. P. LoGerfo. 1981. Hospital medical staff organization and quality of care: Results for myocardial infarction and appendectomy. Medical Care 19(October):1041–1056.

Showstack, A., K. E. Rosenfeld, D. W. Garnick, H. S. Luft, R. W. Schaffarzick, and J. Fowles. 1987. Association of volume with outcome of coronary artery bypass graft surgery. Journal of the American Medical Association (February) 257(6):785–789.

Thomas, L. 1983. The Youngest Science: Notes of a Medicine-Watcher. New York: Viking.

Thomas, L. 1984. Making science work. Pp. 18–28 *in* Late Night Thoughts on Listening to Mahler's Ninth Symphony. New York: Bantam Books.

Perspectives of Industry, the Physician, and Government

Responsibility, Risk, and Informed Consent

PETER F. CARPENTER

Three elements hold the key to the survival and continued success of the biomedical industry in the United States: (1) the way risks are dealt with, both risks of using specific biomedical products and risks associated with innovation of biomedical products in general; (2) the responsibilities of manufacturers, regulators, and users of medical devices and health care products; and (3) the need for the informed consent of the medical device user.

HOW WE DEAL WITH RISK

The problems of product liability in our industry—specifically, those relating to the tort system—have attracted much attention. Unfortunately, because tort law is concerned only with segments of the health care system that fail, our attention has been inappropriately diverted from the much more important objective of achieving success.

The overall quality of medical care and biomedical products has not decreased; significant advances in the pharmaceutical, medical device, and health care arenas continue to occur. Each advance, however, brings with it new risks. Ignoring or refusing to acknowledge these risks as challenges would severely impair our ability to continue to innovate within the health care environment.

The views expressed in this paper are those of the author and not necessarily those of ALZA Corporation or of the biomedical products industry.

We must first acknowledge the impossibility of totally eliminating risk. As von Wartburg (1984) observed:

A fact which is often overlooked is that although the use of certain agents may involve a risk, their non-use is also fraught with problems. While we run the risk of breathing in toxic substances with the air, we are faced with the certain prospect of suffocation if we decide to stop breathing.

Because the biomedical industry deals with issues that affect life and death, we are subject to close scrutiny by the public. Therefore, we must seek creative ways to educate the public and users of our products about risks and benefits. Although risk/benefit assessment has been used extensively in the evaluation of drugs and medical devices, much remains to be done to ensure a better public understanding of the delicate balance between risks and benefits (Carpenter, 1983). For example, if manufacturers more readily acknowledged the possibility of failure of a medical device, then all parties would be better informed and less likely to be surprised when a failure occurs. Manufacturers can also work to minimize the possibility of product failure both by innovative design and labeling.

As organizations and individuals who have voluntarily chosen to participate in the medical marketplace in pursuit of profit, we can never forget that our first responsibility is to those who use our products. We must aim to enhance the quality of their care and to do them no avoidable harm.

RESPONSIBILITIES IN THE HEALTH CARE ARENA

Every participant in the health care arena—manufacturer, doctor, patient, regulator, lawyer, and judge—has special responsibilities. For the United States to retain its position as one of the most medically advanced countries in the world, it is essential that we not only understand but also take these responsibilities seriously.

The responsibilities of the developer and manufacturer are to develop, test, manufacture, and market products that are safe and effective. An important goal during the research and design phase is to reduce unavoidable risks to a minimum. During testing, developers and manufacturers work to expose any previously unknown risks and to reduce them. At the premarket phase, a new biomedical product is usually tested within a small and well-defined set of healthy volunteers and patient subjects. When approved, the product is marketed with a package insert which identifies the product, its indications for use, its benefits, and the known risks associated with its use.

At this point, with necessarily limited experience, the known serious risks are generally few. However, as the product is prescribed for and used by a much larger, more varied, and less controlled patient population, unexpected developments may occur, and manufacturers continue to learn. What is learned about any serious new risk should quickly be reflected in revised labeling. The process of label revision in itself creates an additional legal risk for manufacturers by flagging new concerns that attract the attention of product liability lawyers. At least one major company has gone bankrupt because revision of the label on one of its minor products set the stage for a liability disaster. We must find a way to reduce the adverse impact of this phenomenon so that manufacturers are not discouraged from making timely changes in their labeling.

In communicating all the known benefits and risks to the doctor, we must make clear what type of patient is an appropriate candidate for the product. We have a responsibility not to promote or encourage its use for patients or indications for which it has not been tested or for which the risks outweigh the benefits.

It is the doctor's responsibility to learn everything he or she can about the product. This involves obtaining and becoming familiar with information from the manufacturer, as well as questioning other doctors to learn about their experiences. When prescribing the product, the physician has a crucial responsibility to communicate the potential benefits and risks to the patient. Patients must be told of the possible side effects so that they know what to be alert for.

The informed patient, after leaving the doctor's office, has responsibility for the proper administration and care of the product, as well as for being alert to possible side effects or product failure. If side effects or product failure occurs, the patient is responsible for seeking medical advice quickly.

Follow-up, especially during the initial marketing of a new product, is essential. The doctor, assisted by the patient, must take responsibility for alerting the manufacturer and the Food and Drug Administration (FDA) to any problems experienced with the product.

The United States is behind many other countries in requiring follow-up reporting. Although manufacturers face strict reporting requirements, they must depend on voluntary reports from doctors to alert them or the FDA to problems that patients experience with biomedical products. The United Kingdom's more formalized yellow-card program facilitates adverse reaction reporting by physicians. Although a similar program has been considered here, little progress has been made.

Such a program would be in the best interests of both patients and manufacturers. Good, voluntary, postmarketing surveillance programs may well be the only protection against inappropriate product withdrawals. Such withdrawals will continue to occur in the absence of adequate in-use information. In addition, properly designed postmarketing surveillance programs could provide a competitive advantage for U.S. manufacturing.

INFORMED CONSENT

Jonsen et al. (1982) defines informed consent particularly well:

> Informed consent is defined as the willing and uncoerced acceptance of a medical intervention by a patient after adequate disclosure by the physician of the nature of the intervention, its risks and benefits, as well as of the alternatives with their risks and benefits.

There is a strong tradition in clinical trials and for many surgical procedures of making sure that the participants or patients are well informed about the risks and benefits of the planned medical intervention, and that the participant has freely elected to accept these risks. For some reason this tradition has, in general, not carried over to the postapproval use of most biomedical products. Clearly, such procedures enhance patients' autonomy (Faden and Beauchamp, 1986) by increasing their ability to voluntarily accept or reject risks on a rational basis. It is thus difficult to understand why informed consent is any less important for a patient than for a clinical trial subject.

We live in an age and a country where patients are increasingly interested in and knowledgeable about medical care. Over the past decade, we have seen a dramatic increase in news coverage of medical developments. Gone are the days when patients gave doctors carte blanche to diagnose and treat their ailments. Today, patients are asking informed questions and demanding answers. Perhaps to some physicians, patients who question every aspect of their treatment are an annoyance, but we must remember that patients have both the right and the responsibility to understand their treatment.

Too often we forget that most patients are capable of making knowledgeable decisions. We should take advantage of their increased interest in their medical care to ensure that they are fully aware of risks and benefits. Such awareness should enable a patient to help determine whether he or she is an appropriate candidate for the use of a particular medical product.

Only when the patient or physician believes that the patient has been avoidably harmed by a product should the question of legal liability enter the picture. Today, lawyers have a responsibility not only to their clients but also to the future of health care in this country. Before filing a lawsuit, a lawyer must be relentless in determining probable fault. While I acknowledge lawyers' primary interests must be the protection of their clients, they must also realize that a decision to pursue an inappropriate product liability case in court may have ramifications for the long-term provision of quality health care. The following questions may be appropriately asked: Did the manufacturer mislead the doctor by purposefully concealing a known risk? Did the doctor neglect his or her responsibility to alert the patient to possible serious side effects? Did the patient, having been advised what to look out for, wait too long before seeking medical attention?

Today, manufacturers are caught in a bind. We must pursue innovation in order to improve medical treatment—inventing new devices, developing new drugs, and seeking new uses for and forms of delivery of old drugs. Yet, the threat of product liability hangs over any innovation. This threat provides a powerful motivation for doing everything we can to ensure that medical products and treatments are safe. But that reason should never be the only—or the most important—reason for our commitment to excellence.

Let me illustrate this dichotomy through our recent experience at ALZA Corporation. ALZA is manufacturing and marketing the only intrauterine device (IUD) remaining on the U.S. market. Whether the other manufacturers overreacted by withdrawing their products is a question I cannot answer. I can say, however, that ALZA did not easily reach its decision to keep its IUD on the market.

We immediately recognized that sales of ALZA's IUD, which then had only a very small market share, could dramatically increase. We were concerned that inappropriate use might accompany a marked and uncontrolled increase in use, so our first action was to immediately limit the availability of the IUD Progestasert System to only those physicians who were currently prescribing it, while we assessed the risk factors involved in expanding use of the Progestasert IUD. For example, ALZA conducted detailed reassessment of the new legal risks created by the changed marketing environment.

The Progestasert system is a hormone-releasing IUD that is different in a number of respects from copper-releasing or inert IUDs. When used properly, it is a safe and effective form of birth control. As with all other birth control methods, there are some women for whom the IUD is not appropriate—but does that mean that the option of using an IUD should be taken away from all women, particularly if the IUD has been well designed, tested, manufactured, and labeled to assist proper use?

As part of our decision-making process, ALZA representatives spoke to the people who would be directly and indirectly impacted by our decision. We spoke to women, doctors, consumer advocates, women's health groups, family planning advisers, lawyers, and insurance experts. The objective of this broad consultative process was to increase our understanding of the attitudes and preferences of the groups that our decision would affect. At the same time it provided us with an opportunity to discuss with them some of the considerations involved. To get a balanced perspective, ALZA representatives spoke not only with proponents of birth control but also with individuals and groups who historically have been critical of our product or of IUDs generally.

It did not take long to determine that women and their physicians wanted the option of an IUD—provided that it was properly presented and accurately labeled and that they were given the opportunity to make an informed choice. For example, among women unable to use the birth control pill, the total elimination of the IUD from the market would increase the possibility of unwanted pregnancies—pregnancy is not riskfree. While ALZA realized that keeping its product on the market could be risking lawsuits, it also felt that arbitrarily withdrawing would simply be irresponsible.

Having made the decision to keep our IUD on the market, we were, of course, concerned that the product be used only by appropriate women. And we decided we could help promote this aim further by providing the doctor and patient with updated and expanded information. To do this we developed unusually comprehensive labeling, including an extensive patient information leaflet (*Physicians' Desk Reference*, 1988, pp. 594–596) modeled on the informed consent used for clinical trials.

The leaflet informs the prospective user in detail of known risks and efficacy of the IUD; its format requires the patient's initials at the end of each section to indicate that she has read and understood the information and has discussed her questions with the physician. Although the patient and her doctor may need 30 minutes to go through the leaflet, this is a small investment of time for an important medical decision.

So, for the time being at least, women in the United States still have the option of using an IUD. And, equally importantly, they receive the information necessary to make an informed decision about its use (Medawar, 1986).

A PERSPECTIVE ON FUTURE CHALLENGES

Although the process of deciding whether or not to keep the Progestasert system on the market was long and difficult, I believe we at ALZA have come away with a more enlightened view of the challenges now facing the medical products industry and health care providers. That industry needs to better understand that it does more than simply provide devices or drugs, and that its responsibility does not end when a product goes on the market.

At ALZA, we believe that a biomedical product is much like a piece of computer hardware that requires software to do its job (Mintz, 1987). In the medical arena, the software is every type of information and mechanism that is produced to inform and encourage doctors and patients to use our products correctly. Packaging provides an example, such as the calendar pack used for birth control pills, which is designed to assist patient compliance.

At ALZA, once we determine that a medical product is safe and effective in controlled clinical trials, we ask how we can support its safe and appropriate postapproval use with the proper software. Throughout the medical device industry, such biomedical product software deserves much more attention. It is an area clearly ripe for innovation and as deserving of research investment as the hardware component, which has dominated the industry's research and development programs to date.

In summary, I believe we must dramatically increase public understanding of the inherent risks involved in the use of biomedical products and in biomedical innovation. Only thus can we ensure that all of us are not inappropriately denied the benefits of such products and innovation.

I am not advocating new regulatory solutions. Instead, I believe that smart companies will develop their own creative and innovative software solutions. While the problems with our tort system may take years—maybe even decades—to solve, those of us in the medical products industry can act now. Better product design and testing, better understanding of unavoidable risks, better communication with our product users in the spirit of informed consent regarding the risks, and more timely and compassionate response in the event of unavoidable injury will substantially reduce the opportunities for the tort system to intervene or impede innovation.

The biomedical industry, however, cannot solve all the problems. We must all take it upon ourselves—manufacturers, doctors, lawyers, and patients—to recognize our individual risks and responsibilities and to respond more creatively to the challenges that they pose. We should do it now.

REFERENCES

Carpenter, P. F. 1983. Understanding risk. Medical Device and Diagnostic Industry 5(6):24–26.

Faden, R. R., and T. L. Beauchamp. 1986. P. 8 in Informed Consent. New York: Oxford University Press.

Jonsen, A. R., M. Siegler, and W. J. Winslade. 1982. Clinical Ethics: A Practical Approach to Ethical Decisions in Clinical Medicine. New York: Macmillan.
Medawar, C. 1986. No news, good news? Scrip No. 1162 (December 10):18.
Mintz, M. March 15, 1987. The Washington Post. H6.
Physicians' Desk Reference. 1988. Oradell, N.J.: Medical Economics Company, Inc.
Von Wartburg, W. P. 1984. Drugs and the perception of risks. Swiss Pharma 6(11a):21–23.

The Perspective of the Medical Device Industry

FRANK E. SAMUEL, JR.

TEN STAGES IN THE INNOVATION OF MEDICAL DEVICES

There are ten stages through which medical innovation should flow if we are going to have the highest degree of patient care. Cutting across these stages, there are six factors that can affect the speed and efficiency of the whole process.

My thesis is that we need an integrated approach to policies affecting the invention, development, and use of medical technology. We must not be misled into thinking that simply permitting motivated, self-confident inventors to get a new product into actual use will guarantee success. A fertile invention and prompt development of the product are not enough to assure the best clinical use and appropriate financial treatment for a new medical device. I agree with Edward Roberts (this volume) who said much innovation in health care is neither radical nor research-based, but rather incremental and engineering/development-based. Such innovation takes place every day, through interactions among companies, users, and others. We cannot understand the totality of that process by relying on details surrounding the signal inventions of individuals such as William Greatbatch or Edwin Whitehead.

I also want to point out that it is very difficult to generalize in a useful way about medical technology. Observations based on one technology—even if they are correct—may not apply to pacemakers, patient monitoring equipment, disposable supplies, or other products.

I will only briefly mention the first four stages because they are relatively unaffected by policy decisions of the federal government. These include, first, the discovery of new knowledge; second, awareness of that new knowledge by researchers, clinicians, engineers, and others who can translate the new knowledge into the third stage, invention of a new product; and fourth, patenting the new product. We cannot worry very effectively about the discovery of new knowledge, the invention of new products, or the patenting of new products because I believe that it is the obsessive personal commitment to solving problems by inventing new solutions that drives these steps in the process. I do not believe there is much we can do to encourage that commitment except to continue to protect the values of originality and creativity that our society considers important.

With respect to the second stage, however, there is something to be done. We can work to increase awareness of new knowledge among all people who might play a role in either inventing a new product or in incrementally improving one that is already on the marketplace. The more interchange there is between people doing research and people who have interests in products derived from research the better. As cost constraints continue to be imposed on the health care system, we should increasingly be concerned with the effectiveness and the efficiency of the process by which new technology is transferred from the inventor/scientist to the manufacturer.

The fifth stage in the innovation process is the development of a replicable product, moving from a prototype to a product that can be manufactured in 10, 15, or 100,000 copies; sent into the field; used in institutions by a wide variety of people; and perform the way it was intended to perform. That step in innovation is extremely important; yet it is difficult, time-consuming, and unpredictable. It is a step that policymakers are inclined to ignore, believing that all it takes is a workable prototype to be able to translate a new technology into dependable patient care.

In the sixth stage, a clinical trial is conducted, the results of which will be used to acquire Food and Drug Administration (FDA) approval of the new product.

These stages, however, are neither rigidly sequential nor performed in mutually exclusive time frames. They are not neat. The development of a replicable medical device and the conduct of a clinical trial may go hand in hand, and it is important to remember that much interactive development of new devices takes place.

The seventh stage in the innovation process is obtaining FDA approval based on the results of the clinical trial and other relevant information.

Once FDA approval has been obtained, coverage and payment decisions must be made by various health care insurance and government programs. This is the eighth step. Although we are often preoccupied with federal programs such as Medicare, we must remember that Medicare pays only 40 percent of hospital costs; 60 percent is paid by Blue Cross and other private insurers. Here, therefore, nongovernmental decisions, whether or not they are made thoughtfully or by default, are at least as important as governmental decisions.

It is particularly unfortunate that the courts and Congress are deciding issues about the coverage of new medical technologies. There ought to be an effective nonpolitical way to adjust the systems for financing health care that take account of specific new technologies. But as Stuart Altman has explained (this volume), we may not be doing a very good job of this; if we are not, then the courts and Congress will continue to be used as agents of last resort.

The ninth and tenth stages are generally underemphasized, but I believe we will hear more about them in the future. Stage nine is postmarketing surveillance by the FDA, and stage ten is postcoverage review by insurance companies.

Technology manufacturers have always been sensitive to the issue of postmarketing review because it sounds like additional regulatory requirements. There is already, on average, a 13-month delay after the clinical trial for new medical devices that must be approved by the FDA. Suggesting that FDA ought to do postmarketing surveillance after all this premarketing review has always seemed an additional burden for manufacturers aimed not at improving health care, but at protecting the reputation of the regulators.

However, if we are going to ask for faster market introduction of certain kinds of technologies or for interim coverages for those technologies that were mentioned by Seymour Perry (this volume), then manufacturers should be willing to recognize that clinical data-based postmarketing surveillance may become necessary.

Manufacturers must also assume that, as health care providers and third-party payers become increasingly concerned with cost-containment, they will begin to look for "obsolete" medical technologies, including both procedures and products. To this end, stages nine and ten can play an important role in determining the appropriate use of medical technologies.

These, then, are the ten stages in the innovation of new medical devices. Innovative products do not move consecutively or with uniformity of speed through those stages, of course. But at each stage, different actors and factors play key roles; we would lose some important distinctions if we attempt to compress the innovative process into fewer stages.

FACTORS INFLUENCING THE TEN STAGES
IN MEDICAL DEVICE INNOVATION

An issue that cuts across several of these stages is professional and patient acceptance of new medical technologies. Professional acceptance in particular used to be the major factor necessary for successful innovation in health care; today, however, it is one of many important factors.

Both product liability and issues of corporate research and development taxation are also important. The suggestion made by Susan Bartlett Foote (this volume) to make compensation for injury fair and more predictable by separating compensation decisions from issues of generalized product liability was very constructive.

International competition in medical devices is important, and it affects different segments of the industry to different extents. For example, international competition in capital equipment manufacturing is much greater than it is for supplies used in hospitals.

Ethical considerations in health care, particularly with respect to patients who have terminal diseases or who are otherwise vulnerable, will become increasingly important. The final factor that bears on several stages of medical innovation is the availability of funds for research, product development, regulation, and services. In the area of services, payments for medical care provided to the uninsured, for long-term care, and for some new procedures that can be performed outside hospitals are currently underfunded.

The Health Industry Manufacturers Association (HIMA) has paid much attention to the availability of funds for regulation in the last couple of years, because regulation delayed is product improvement delayed and patient care improvement denied.

The spirit of our health care system is to improve delivered care. We must therefore have a regulatory process that dependably, reliably, and credibly enables and promotes that process. The regulatory process for medical devices should not just deter bad things from happening, it should have the positive value of ensuring that better things continue to happen. That does not necessarily mean that it is desirable that devices go through the FDA approval process in 5 or 6 months instead of 12 months.

The point is that the movement of devices through the system should be both swift and credible. The public benefits from having such a regulatory process; industry also benefits from having a credible process. It does the industry no good to have medical devices reviewed for safety and efficacy by regulators who are poorly trained. A regulatory agency should be staffed with professionals who are cognizant of the state of the art of medical technologies. Both the public and the medical devices industry will rely on decisions made by such an agency, but we are not at that point.

To support such changes, HIMA has recommended higher appropriations for the FDA. HIMA's argument, stated again, is that regulation delayed is product improvements delayed and patient care improvements denied. HIMA's position reinforces and supports the fundamental impulse of health care, which is not only to avoid bad outcomes but to make things better.

Are any of these ten stages or any of the factors influencing them becoming simpler, less expensive, or more predictable? No. In general, the overall process is becoming more expensive and less predictable, although it is hard to pinpoint exactly what stages and factors are responsible for this change. The process is becoming more expensive and less predictable, in part because we have more government involvement in the health care system. Also, insurance systems are, for the first time, taking a role in technology assessment, and in part, innovation of medical devices is becoming more complicated and less predictable because many medical devices are interacting in a more complex way with the human body. Such a change may require a level of expertise that is difficult to achieve and results that are difficult to regulate.

SOME SUGGESTIONS FOR CHANGE

First, we need to explore ways to enhance the transfer of new technology. The National Academy of Engineering and the Institute of Medicine should continue to work together to enhance communication about medical device innovation across disciplinary lines. Leo Thomas (this volume) emphasizes the value of an interdisciplinary approach, and I believe he is correct. New medical technologies will come from advances in materials science, electronics, and related activities, as well as from biological and clinical research.

A second important area is user education. If we want to have a quick impact on the quality of care in the United States, we should put aside changes in products. Instead, we should concentrate on ensuring that the products are used the way they were intended to be used. Whether health care providers follow reasonable standards in reuse of disposable products or acceptable procedures for calibrating anesthesiology equipment, the single greatest opportunity for short-term improvements in patient care remains greater education for the users of medical devices.

No single entity or group can achieve that goal. Professional groups, hospital administrators, and biomedical engineers must all be involved. Clearly, device manufacturers, the FDA, and the Health Care Financing Administration are involved. And not least important, the federal government should designate a modest amount of money for training or retraining health care providers.

My third recommendation concerns product liability. Some of the suggestions made by Susan Bartlett Foote (this volume) are constructive and appropriately focused on health care. Instead of dealing separately with professional, hospital, and other facility malpractice and product liability for medical device manufacturers that grow out of a single incident of injury to a patient, all claims should be considered together, not piecemeal.

Fourth, we all need to think seriously about what quality health care means. In part, it is a question of data collection; in part, it is a question of coming to grips with measures of outcomes. Frankly, the notion of quality has become devalued and empty of meaning in policy circles because it is seen as a buzz word that providers and suppliers use to protect themselves. But quality does not mean whatever we want it to mean. It cannot mean more tax shelters for physicians, more diversification for hospitals, and more expensive product refinements for manufacturers. Quality must be given meaning in relation to patient care.

Fifth, I believe we are facing a significant issue in funding for clinical trials. For 20 years, Medicare has taken the position that it has no responsibility to fund clinical trials for new drugs or devices. Experimental, investigational technologies are not "reasonable and necessary." This means that Medicare takes no responsibility for improving the health of Medicare beneficiaries.

Now, this position is not a question of law; the Medicare statute does not require it. I think that is an unreasonable policy, and one that the Institute of Medicine should explore.

Sixth, and last, we need to look at the technology of long-term care: where it is delivered, who delivers it, quality controls for long-term care, and so forth. In an era dominated by AIDS and an aging population, it is a topic that is going to demand the best from all of us.

Prospective Payment

HARVEY V. FINEBERG

What is, perhaps, most important about the Prospective Payment System is that prospective payment represents a more centrally controllable pattern of payment for health care services than did cost-based reimbursement.

As we consider moving from the Prospective Payment System, which is payment based on episode of illness, to payment systems such as capitation and other systems of managed care, the effect will be to further enhance centralized control of such decisions as how much is going to be spent and where it is going to be spent. Centralization of such decisions may have an impact on the availability of new medical devices.

What the current system introduces is uncertainty about those effects. One of the key features that needs to be incorporated into the thinking of the Prospective Payment Commission, Medicare program administrators, and all those who have some control over the payment system, is increasing the assurance about the way in which payments will be made over a period of time. Such assurance will enhance stability in planning and projection throughout the whole system.

We will inevitably see an increasing investment in health care in this country. The pressures of an aging population, of rising income in the population, and of new disease problems all point in that direction. Will we be able to allocate effectively the resources that must pay for these services in this era of centralized decision making? The answer depends on how much money we put into the Prospective Payment System and how it is directed to be spent.

In the future, physicians increasingly will be subject to the incentives of prospective payment. The growth in prepayment for services and in the number of physicians that are salaried instead of working as free-standing entrepreneurs—a trend which is almost sure to continue—alters the financial incentives that the physician sees. That, combined with the traditional role of the physician as decision maker about adoption and use of new medical devices and technologies, will have a bearing on some segments of the medical device industry over time.

Today, for example, the practice of performing medical tests in the physician's office is growing at a rate of about 16 to 19 percent per year, double the rate of growth of hospital-based or independent laboratory testing. This change is partly driven by advances in technology and the capacity to do more in the office. It is also driven, in part, by recent changes in reimbursement: Whereas hospital-based tests are part of a diagnosis-related group and subject to the constraints of prospective payment, office-based tests are not. The kinds of incentives that differentially affect specific segments are likely to continue and change.

REGULATION AND PRODUCT LIABILITY

The new tensions between the objectives of the regulatory system and the liability system that have been addressed by Susan Bartlett Foote in her contribution to this volume are very important. The key piece of information that would permit us to move toward a reasonable system for compensation, and which is missing, is information on the frequency and severity of medical events that have negative outcomes for patients. It is going to be very hard to adopt a program that automatically compensates patients for bad outcomes when we do not have good data about the frequency and severity of these outcomes.

BIOMEDICAL INNOVATION

Several individuals have suggested that the United States needs to have an explicit strategy to promote biomedical innovation in research, in the field, and in industry; that we do need to think about biomedical innovation systematically; and that we should be seeking ways to encourage the kind of creativity, inventiveness, and independence that seem to be at the heart of successful innovation in the past. Several approaches have been suggested: various industry/university associations, the kind of small business investment program that the National Institutes of Health has started, the possibility of consortia funded or convened under government auspices, and various proposals for coordinating and integrating interagency activities within the government.

At the same time, others have stressed that such early stages of creativity and innovation are characterized by individual initiative and will proceed regardless of what we do; these stages do not need to be stimulated.

I propose that we have an experimental attitude toward stimulating innovation. And we should develop concrete suggestions for ways in which we retrospectively can decide what experiments have worked and what has enhanced our capacity for innovation. The net effects of the current uncertainty about future payment systems and the medical device industry act to dampen attention to and investment in medical progress.

EVALUATING MEDICAL DEVICES

It is important to distinguish between decisions to make available medical devices and decisions to actually use the devices. What is most important is not whether a device is good or bad once it has passed the hurdles of industry assessment and Food and Drug Administration assessment, but how well it is being used in the medical community. To evaluate a device, then, it is not sensible to evaluate only the device per se, but rather to think about the system in which the device is employed. Such an evaluation must consider the particular patient population subjected to the device; the particular setting in which the device is used (hospital, clinic, or home); and the providers involved (physicians, technicians, and others). The system applied to the evaluation of each device will be specific to these and other circumstances.

Much of that is behind concerns over misapplication of devices or technology; not that they are good or bad, but that they may be used in varying beneficial and risky ways. For example, our own studies of computed tomography (CT) scanning at a major teaching hospital have demonstrated more than a sixfold difference in the frequency with which use of the CT scan affected treatment decisions for different classes of patients.

In a recent assessment of thrombolytic treatment of patients who have a myocardial infarction, taking into consideration only the size of the infarction and how soon after the infarction the patient arrives in the emergency room, there was at least a 10-fold difference in the costs of having one more patient alive at the end of 1 year. From the point of view of physicians in practice, decisions about good technologies—how they are used, when they are used, in what patients they are used—are at the crux of the evaluation problem.

Additionally, all evaluation is relative to some alternative. Susan Foote discussed the risks of allowing judgments about the appropriateness of medical devices to be made in court, and I agree that it is unlikely to be effective. But we should recognize that if those judgments are to be made by physicians and evaluators in an informed way, they must also be made relative to the alternatives. There is always the alternative of not doing anything for the patient, and there are likely to be alternative interventions for each patient.

It is important to remember that having a good device and having a complete evaluation that assesses the effectiveness of that device does not guarantee that the device will be used as it has been evaluated. It takes time for good devices, properly used, to diffuse and disseminate into practice. Factors that influence diffusion and use of new devices and other medical technology raise important issues that, if properly addressed, will improve the way in which medical care is delivered and the cost sensitivity of that care.

Finally, I offer a reminder. All research directed toward innovation for medical devices and, more broadly, toward innovation in health care is aimed at a future benefit. We are, in effect, deferring current consumption and current use of resources to invest in the development of improved future health care. If we keep in mind the goal of improving the health of particular patients or groups of patients in the future, it is incumbent upon us also to think broadly about the role of technology in enhancing the health of people over time and strategically about how we can move our health care system in those directions.

For example, there are about 15 countries that have lower infant mortality rates than the United States. What is our problem? Ounce for ounce, we do as well as any country in the world; we save more infants of low birth weight than any other country in the world. Our problem is that we have too many low-birth-weight infants. If we are going to decrease our infant mortality rate, we must think critically about how to reduce the frequency of low birth weight; this is a very different problem than how well we can keep a 550-gram infant alive.

If our goal is to keep the number of people who die from heart disease at a minimum in the year 2010, how do we get to that goal? We have made remarkable progress against heart disease in the last 25 years; since the late 1960s, the incidence of heart disease as a cause of death has been steadily declining in the United States. Most of the decline is because fewer people are having heart attacks: Diet has changed; we have improved treatment of hypertension; tobacco use has declined; we have improved the care of patients after they have heart attacks. Thinking ahead, we should ask ourselves how we can take advantage of what we know today so that people who would otherwise be dead or incapacitated from heart attacks will be alive in the year 2010.

A final example is the issue of injury from automobile accidents. Why do we have a problem? Because we do not yet adequately protect the occupants of automobiles, we do not have appropriate policies to deal with the problemn of driving while intoxicated, and we do not invest enough in road safety (lighted roads and better markings) to reduce the frequency of severe and disabling accidents.

How Trends Will Interact:
The Perspective of the Government

LOUISE B. RUSSELL

The government has at least four major perspectives on new medical devices in health care. First, it is a major funder of research. Second, it is a major financer of care. Third, the government serves as guardian of the public interest; that is, it protects the safety of the public and tries to ensure fair dealing. Each of these activities is conducted through different agencies—for example, financing of care through the

Health Care Financing Administration, financing of research through the National Institutes of Health, and guarding of the public interest through the Food and Drug Administration and the Federal Trade Commission. And there are other agencies involved in these activities.

The fourth perspective of the government comes from a responsibility that encompasses all of these: The government provides a forum for the resolution of conflicting interests. The Congress and the judicial system, more than the executive branch agencies, provide this forum. Private interests are reconciled when private conflicts are brought to the government's attention. But the government's different roles—its different perspectives—also produce conflicts that must be reconciled. Thus, the government has the additional job of reconciling its different roles to reflect the public interest.

Reading the inventors' stories contained in this volume, I was struck by the breadth of time they covered—from World War II to the present day—and by how much the government's roles from each of the four perspectives has changed during that time. Government has both made the trends and responded to them. Its actions also refer to other trends beyond those considered here, trends in the larger economy and in domestic and world events. I will review the changes in the government's roles in medical device innovation during the last 35 years; this will provide the background for projecting changes in the government's roles in the future.

THE GOVERNMENT'S ROLE IN RESEARCH

The 1950s and 1960s were halcyon days for medical research. National spending on health research and development more than quadrupled from 0.06 percent of the gross national product (GNP) in 1950 to 0.27 percent in 1970 (National Institutes of Health, 1975; U.S. Bureau of the Census, 1985). The nation's economic resources were growing, and an increasing share of those resources was being allotted to medical research.

Responding to the wealth of new possibilities in medical research and the public's desire to benefit from those possibilities, the federal government became a major player in medical research. By 1970, the National Institutes of Health (NIH) dominated the federal role in supporting medical research. NIH's share of all health research and development (R&D) dollars rose from less than 20 percent in 1950 to about 40 percent in 1970 (National Institutes of Health, 1975). Since then, national spending on health research and development has leveled off at about 0.30 percent of the GNP, and NIH still accounted for

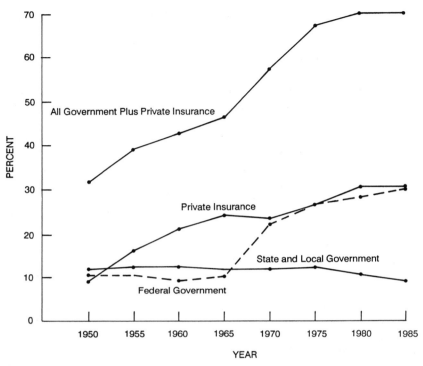

FIGURE 1   Third-party payment for medical care.

about 40 percent of the total in 1985 (National Institutes of Health, 1985; U.S. Bureau of Economic Analysis, 1987).

THE GOVERNMENT'S ROLE IN FINANCING HEALTH CARE

Third-party payment for medical care by private insurers and the government has grown enormously since 1950 (Figure 1) (U.S. Social Security Administration, 1976; Waldo et al., 1986). In the beginning, the government was primarily an observer; many federal programs were debated, but few were passed. Meanwhile, private insurance payments rose from less than 10 percent of total expenditures for personal health care in 1950 to nearly 25 percent in 1965. During these years, health care spending by federal programs remained at about 10 percent of the total, and state and local spending remained at about 12 percent.

With the passage of Medicare and Medicaid, the federal government took a much larger role in financing health care—its share of expenditures for personal health care rose to 22 percent in 1970 and gradually increased to its current 30 percent. Private insurance payments also continued to grow and are now about 30 percent, while state and local government spending has declined slightly, to less than 10 percent of the total. State and local governments, however, have control over more money than this figure indicates since they are responsible for allocating some federal funds, especially the matching funds provided for Medicaid.

These changes have radically altered the market for medical services. Third-party payment covered 30 percent of expenditures for personal health care in 1950, increased to 70 percent by 1980, and remained at that level in 1985. More money for research brought a host of new technologies that could save lives and improve health. More money for health care services made it possible for most people to avail themselves of these technologies, as when Medicare was extended to pay the costs of dialysis for people with end-stage renal disease.

THE GOVERNMENT AS GUARDIAN OF THE PUBLIC INTEREST

The government's role as guardian of the public interest and public safety has also expanded. Government regulation of medical devices expanded under the Medical Device Amendments of 1976. The Food and Drug Administration's responsibility for drugs has been widened to include efficacy as well as safety. Health care services have been increasingly regulated through health planning, certificate of need, professional standards review organizations (PSROs), and PSROs' successors, the professional review organizations.

In addition, the government is involved in the growth of medical liability cases through state and federal court systems and through state oversight of health insurance companies.

THE STAGE IS SET

These three trends—research, financing, and regulation—have converged in recent years; in each case, growth has leveled off after a period of rapid increases and major change. As a percentage of the GNP, federal spending on research has been stable for more than 10 years. Spending on health care services by all levels of government has been a stable percentage of spending on all services for nearly as long—federal spending has crept up a few points, but state and local spending has declined. The Medical Device Amendments are still not fully implemented. Health planning has been repealed.

The leveling off has occurred for two reasons. One is that the nation's resource base has not grown as fast as it did earlier. The GNP per civilian worker, corrected for inflation, has grown much more slowly in the last 15 years than it did in the two decades ending in 1970 (calculated from the Economic Report of the President, 1986).

The second reason is that no sector can increase its share of the national pie forever—the enormous growth enjoyed by medical research and medical services in the 1950s and 1960s, and even a little beyond, had to end sometime. For the last several years (longer for research), government spending on health care has grown as fast as the GNP, but not faster. The combination of a stable share and a more slowly growing GNP has meant considerably slower growth for the medical sector. Total national health expenditures have remained at just over 10.5 percent of the GNP since 1982 (Waldo et al., 1986).

I project that this situation will continue for some time, unlike earlier periods when health spending leveled off for a couple of years before increasing again. This means that, while the market for medical devices is large and will remain large, it will not grow faster than the GNP. Unless the GNP grows faster than it has in the past 5 or 10 years, growth in the market for medical devices will be rather slow.

A bright spot, however, is offered by the recent fall in the value of the dollar relative to currencies of other countries. By February 1985, compared with the currencies of our major trading partners, the dollar had risen 81 percent above the average level of 1980 (Board of Governors, Federal Reserve System, 1987). In the last 2 years it has fallen until it is nearly back to the level of 1980. The higher dollar made it difficult for U.S. producers of anything—medical devices included—to compete with foreign producers and encouraged production abroad. The recent fall of the dollar greatly improves the ability of medical device manufacturers to sell their products to other countries. Better markets abroad should help counter the change in growth of domestic markets, and could also provide a rationale for increased investments by the private sector.

THE GOVERNMENT AS RECONCILER OF CONFLICTING INTERESTS, INCLUDING ITS OWN

I have projected that government spending on health, whether for research or services, will not grow very much as a percentage of the GNP in the next few years. Indeed, I suspect that total spending—private as well as government—will not grow much. In the future, there are likely to be shifts of emphasis within the total amount government spends on health, not a decision to change the GNP share for medical care relative to other goods and services. If this is the case, the government will have a difficult role to play reconciling the conflicting interests of those who would like a larger share of the resources pie. It has sampled this new role in the last few years with the implementation of policies like the Prospective Payment System, which were implemented to help slow increases in government expenditures for health care.

For these reasons, I agree with Anthony Romeo's conclusion (this volume) that there is no rationale for increasing federal funding for research at this time. In addition, the large and continuing federal deficits make it unlikely that there will be large increases in any kind of federal spending, medical or nonmedical.

All health care services and all technologies—new and old—are likely to be affected by slower growth in the future. Cost-reducing technologies or services should do better in this new fiscal environment than they did previously since they free resources for other uses. With new resources hard to come by, cost savings will be a valuable source of funds. The effects of the new resource-constrained environment on cost-increasing technologies or services should depend on their benefits relative to their costs. If benefits are high, cost-increasing technologies or services should be used almost as widely as they would have been if health expenditures were growing rapidly. If benefits are low, they should be used with considerably more restraint; if the benefits are low enough, they may not be used at all.

Thus, some new technologies will continue to diffuse rapidly, others will spread more slowly and less extensively than they would have under conditions of rapidly increasing resources for medical care, and some may be cut back. The effects of slow growth will be easiest to spot when technologies or services are cut back; for rapidly diffusing technologies, it will be harder to discern the difference between the old environment and the new one.

There is already some evidence for these responses to slowed growth of resources for medical care. Stuart Altman noted (this volume) that magnetic resonance imaging (MRI) seems to have spread fairly rapidly in spite of the Prospective Payment System (PPS). However, PPS may be one of the reasons MRI has spread more slowly than computed axial tomography (CAT) did, and it is almost certainly one of the reasons that MRI has been located in outpatient settings much more than CAT was (Steinberg et al., 1985). Altman also noted that the new pacemakers, which became available just before prospective payment was introduced, have also been accepted quite rapidly.

At the same time, a study by the General Accounting Office (1986) found that the use of intensive care for Medicare patients dropped after the introduction of prospective payment. The study covered the years 1981 through 1984. From 1981 to 1983 the number of days of intensive care used by Medicare beneficiaries increased every year. Between 1983 and 1984, the first year of prospective payment, the number of days used declined 14 percent.

Reconciling conflicting interests in a situation of slow growth obviously poses many difficult choices. What sorts of policy does this suggest for the future? What sorts of changes will there be in the government role? I suggest three sorts of changes that echo themes sounded by other contributors to this volume. The first is that direct spending is unlikely to be a major method for reconciling conflicts in the future. It will no longer be possible to resolve conflicts by giving some parties more money and letting others keep what they already have; instead, money may have to be shifted from one party to another. The second change is that payment systems will continue to evolve in ways that encourage conflicting interests to achieve their own solutions. The third change is that the need to resolve conflicts will lead—is already leading—to more emphasis on gathering and sharing information.

Changes in the Payment System

The government is already playing an important role in changing the way medical care is paid for and will continue to do so. The direction has been set; the nation will not return to cost-based reimbursement. Future changes will probably take the payment system in the direction of more global prospective payment, toward a system that covers more services, providers, and payers. This will bring budgetary constraints to bear more evenly across the health care system. It also should help avoid some of the peculiar results now appearing as providers move services away from tightly constrained settings and into those that are, for now, less constrained.

It is important to remember that no payment system can be problem-free. No payment system is capable of making everybody happy and of never producing an odd or an unfair result. Further, I submit that there is no such thing as the "neutral" payment system that Stuart Altman has described. For a payment system to be considered neutral, it would have to produce results that everybody agreed were the appropriate ones; there is no consensus on what the best, or appropriate, results are.

Information for Making Choices

Decisions about the adoption and use of new technologies are more difficult in a period of slow growth. Not only the benefits and risks but also the costs of the technology must be weighed, because costs represent the alternatives that must be given up in order to use the technology in question. Such decisions can be described as allocating resources, or rationing resources, or making appropriate use of resources; the terms are interchangeable. The resources available to the medical sector are not sufficient to do everything that everyone would like to do, and some hard decisions must be made about which things will get the most attention.

Information is essential for good decisions, but information is not always welcome. Information makes decisions clearer, and thus more painful. Thus, there will be times when, although it seems sensible to learn as much as possible in order to make the best decision possible, people would really rather not know that much about the implications of their decisions.

As the nation tries to use its medical resources appropriately in the years ahead, those involved in the decisions will ask for more information than they have in the past, notwithstanding the discomfort information sometimes causes. With resources growing slowly, we are more concerned about what we are getting in return for what we are spending. Every actor in the system, including government, will want more information upon which to base its decisions.

I cite two examples of what I see as an increasing appetite for information. The first is the release of hospital mortality data by the Health Care Financing Administration. Mortality is a crude measure of outcome, but the release of these data was a useful step in beginning to focus people's attention on outcomes and the variation in outcomes among providers. Making the data public has started people thinking about how to improve them so that they will more accurately reflect quality of care. The second example is manufacturers' increasing interest in comparing the efficacy of their products with that of competing products. Such information should be valuable to patients as well as to manufacturers and their clients.

Finally, I want to emphasize that when information is created, it should be made available to all the players—not just providers, or manufacturers, or doctors, but to patients as well. Patients have more reason than anyone else to be concerned with the choices made about allocating medical resources. They should have the opportunity to get involved in both national and individual decisions.

POSSIBLE ROLE FOR THE INSTITUTE OF MEDICINE

Frank Samuel (this volume) rightly urged the importance of carefully defining quality of care in terms of outcomes. Cost-containment has brought new attention to this issue because of the fear that pressures to cut costs will lead to reductions in quality and poorer outcomes. In my view, we have been too complacent about quality. Quality deserved more attention before prospective payment, and one of the good results of prospective payment is that quality is receiving more attention now.

A number of organizations are interested in the issue of quality of care. Many of them have undertaken studies. But, except for the Health Care Financing Administration, which for obvious reasons should not be counted on to provide complete and objective information, none of them is in a position to produce more than a series of small, rather specialized studies. A lot of small studies undertaken according to the ideas of each individual group may not add up to very much.

The Institute of Medicine could provide an overall plan—a research agenda—that would allow these organizations to tailor their studies to provide pieces of information that, taken together, would produce a more coherent view of outcomes. The Institute of Medicine is ideally suited to this task for several reasons: It is not tied to any of the major actors—government, providers, insurers, or patients—yet it is a national organization that can call on any of them for advice and help; it has the credibility to get attention for its recommendations; and it brings together in its members all the disciplines that would need to be involved in providing such guidance.

The research agenda should include components ranging from recommendations about methods to monitoring work in the field. It should outline the available methods for studying outcomes and indicate which have been validated. The best methods are likely to be complex and expensive, and the plan could indicate the circumstances in which simpler methods would be useful and circumstances in which only the best would do. The plan could point out issues and groups most in need of detailed study; it could also point out the methodological areas in greatest need of work. The Institute could monitor developments in the field, revising the agenda as necessary. It could also, of course, contribute some of the required studies.

There is no conflict between the short and long term in developing such a plan; the issue of quality is not going to go away. The research agenda would necessarily start with what is going on now, providing an overall framework that made clear the best and worst aspects of current activity. Such a framework would help set the direction for the next decade and beyond.

REFERENCES

Board of Governors of the Federal Reserve System. 1987. Federal Reserve Bulletin 73(2). Washington, D.C.: Federal Reserve System.

General Accounting Office. 1986. Medicare Past Overuse of Intensive Care Services Inflates Hospital Payments. Washington, D.C.: U.S. Government Printing Office.

National Institutes of Health. 1975. Basic Data Relating to the National Institutes of Health. Washington, D.C.: Department of Health, Education, and Welfare.

National Institutes of Health. 1985. Basic Data Book: Basic Data Relating to the National Institutes of Health. Washington, D.C.: Department of Health and Human Services.

Steinberg, E. P., J. E. Sisk, and K. E. Locke. 1985. X-ray CT and magnetic resonance imagers. New England Journal of Medicine 313(14):859–864.

U.S. Bureau of the Census. 1985. Statistical abstract of the United States: 1986, 106th ed. Washington, D.C.: Department of Commerce.

U.S. Bureau of Economic Analysis. 1987. Survey of Current Business 67(1). Washington, D.C., Department of Commerce.

Economic Report of the President. 1986. Washington, D.C.: U.S. Government Printing Office.

U.S. Social Security Administration. 1976. Compendium of National Health Expenditures Data. Compiled by B. S. Cooper, N. L. Worthington, and M. F. McGee. Washington, D.C.: Department of Health, Education, and Welfare.

Waldo, D. R., K. R. Levit, and H. Lazenby. 1986. National health expenditures, 1985. Health Care Financing Review 8(1):1–21.

Summarizing Reflections

WILLIAM W. LOWRANCE

Two general impressions pervade the papers in this volume and my recollections of the symposium on which it is based.* The first is an overwhelming admiration of the medical armamentarium that has become available. What a range of devices now can be drawn upon to measure physiological parameters, to peer right through the body, to deliver drugs precisely, to make surgical and other repairs, to replace tissues and bones and organs, to compensate for sensory and mobility losses, to bolster recovery! So although this volume was conceived and assembled in the interest of encouraging and guiding innovation, we should not feel too bad about the accomplishments so far.

The second impression is a sense that the rubric "medical devices" covers an almost unencompassable range of technologies—from rather simple classical aids, such as crutches and eyeglasses, to novel high-technology instruments and implantable organs, and from inexpensive devices used intimately by individuals, to capital hardware used in large institutions for the benefit of many thousands. This makes the topic exceedingly difficult to analyze as a category, and frustrating to deal with as a policy and legal problem.

Frank Samuel, paraphrasing Gertrude Stein on Oakland, has said of the medical device territory, "There is no there there. . . ."

* "New Medical Devices: Factors Influencing Invention, Development, and Use." Symposium sponsored by the National Academy of Engineering and the Institute of Medicine, March 9–10, 1987, Washington, D.C.

But Frank's own employment as an industry leader is evidence that within the territory, despite its unruliness, addressable issues exist.

SALIENT TRENDS IN HEALTH CARE

The many health care trends covered in the preceding papers need not be reviewed here, but a few with special relevance to the device enterprise are worth noting: *ambulatory care, home care, self-care, noninvasiveness, long-term care,* and *rehabilitation.*

The overarching concerns of everyone in the enterprise are to ensure quality and to preserve the ethical complexion of care, even as costs are being subjected to vigorous campaigns of containment.

Seymour Perry and others make it clear that health care is being monitored and evaluated more systematically than ever before. This is a crucial development, one long overdue. Finally we may learn what the paybacks really are from our personal and social medical investments. But for innovators and providers, having people "looking over their shoulders" and reviewing their billings—institutionalizing *caveat emptor,* so to speak—is unsettling.

THE FLOW OF INNOVATION

The evolution of a technology from conception to full use can be schematized as shown in Figure 1. A new medical device is conceived in a marriage between technical opportunity and medical need. Perhaps more than for some other kinds of technologies, the elements of the medical innovative partnership may be quite distinct, as was implied by the joint sponsorship of the symposium from which this book derives.

Engineers, materials scientists, inventors, systems specialists, and others on the supply side seek beneficial uses for their technologies. Physicians, health care experts, and patient advocates on the demand side seek technologies to meet health needs. The problem is how to explore potential matches between the two sides. In some cases one person competently bridges between these universes. But more often, nowadays, the task requires organized teams.

Following the almost magical step of *innovation*—which may result from a stroke of genius, inspired tinkering, modest improvement of a conventional device, or strategically pursued fancy-technology R&D— a prototype is moved into development.

Development may make variations on the initial invention, then subject prototypes to testing, evaluation, and improvement. Consid-

THE FLOW OF INNOVATION

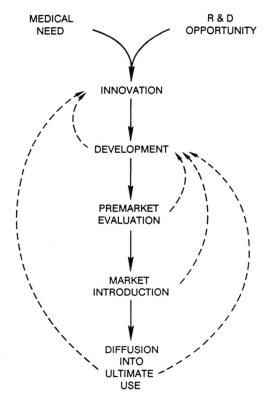

FIGURE 1   The flow of innovation.

eration is given to the pragmatics of manufacture. Consideration also is given to the vagaries of real-world application and use.

If the invention looks promising, it moves on into *premarket evaluation,* being put through carefully staged testing, perhaps on animals first, then on people, to gain realistic assessment of its medical potential. In part because of the enormous diversity of these products, in part because of the intensity of their medical effects, and in part because of the pace and complexity of their design evolution, the choice of criteria by which medical devices should be evaluated is not always clear or fully anticipatable.

If, after all this evaluation, the device still looks medically promising, and looks financially promising to the vendor, and can meet the various government regulatory and other "filtering" standards of efficacy and safety, it is moved into *marketing*.

If the innovation continues to meet all these criteria and its market grows, it undergoes wider *diffusion into ultimate use*. Several substages may have to be passed through before the device becomes fully established.

Figure 1, though an idealized representation, helps to show the flow of innovation and the factors influencing it. For the moment, merely notice the dotted retro-connections indicated by dotted lines. These are feedback loops, a notion that both physicians and engineers are accustomed to. There is feedback between development and initial innovation, and between various later stages and development and innovation. And in the largest picture, there is feedback between both present and potential use and initial innovation.

HEALTH OF THE DEVICE ENTERPRISE ITSELF

A question expressed or implied by all the authors in this collection of papers is: Is the medical-device delivery enterprise itself, as a system, healthy?

For the various reasons cited, it is difficult to generalize. But the external evidence is fairly heartening. Manufacturers are still turning relatively solid profits. Few of them are getting out of the business. Unlike Chrysler, the steel manufacturers, and the railroads, the medical manufacturers—with the exception of a few producers of vaccines or intrauterine devices (IUDs)—have not begged for federal bailout or special treatment. Entrepreneurial investors are still lining up.

Thus for those who invent, develop, and make devices, the outlook seems far from bleak. For all of us who are the ultimate consumers of devices, surely, despite a variety of problems and costs, we have never been better served.

The test questions to this broad issue are: Are any major, promisingly beneficial medical devices being denied to the world because of lack of support for, or impediments to, R&D? Or because of inadequate protection of proprietary rights? Or because of repressive regulation? Or because of the threat from unjustified legal liability? Or because of market failures?

Tentatively—since the authors do not review cases in economic detail—the answer seems to be: no; few, if any, lines of medical technology development have been stifled (with the possible exception of vaccines), although possibly a few have been slowed.

Robert Mann refers to deceleration of R&D. John Moxley says

hospitals are slowing their purchasing of big instruments. From their broad perspective, Samuel Thier and Stuart Altman observe that cost-containment has not substantially retarded *innovation,* though it may have slowed sales and retarded increase in use. Edwin Whitehead and Alan Kahn, speaking as innovators, agree that there has been little damping of important invention. Walter Robb notes that, at least for some large manufacturers, innovation is shifting more to devices that can reduce per-unit care costs, and away from those that offer truly novel kinds of care.

It appears that even for such controversial examples as diagnostic imaging, the industry continues to burgeon. New principles and models keep being introduced, and more and more citizens enjoy access to imaging services.

One clear example of near-extinction of both innovation and use is IUDs. This volume does not discuss the Dalkon Shield lawsuits and related issues, although Susan Bartlett Foote refers to them. Peter Carpenter describes how his firm has gone about marketing its IUD, taking elaborate precautions to inform potential users of benefits and risks and secure informed consent.

If any proposed devices are being orphaned because the potential market for them is small, despite serious medical neediness, their orphan status may be recognized and special support sought for them. Similarly, if any proposed technologies are languishing because of undue legal liability or other impediments, special subsidy or indemnification may be sought; the National Childhood Vaccine Injury Act of 1986 attempts to provide such support (the act was passed but, as of mid-1988, has not been implemented).

Beyond invention, obviously there are barriers to widespread practical adoption. For instance, Seymour Perry and Stuart Altman point out difficulties the Prospective Payment System encounters in accommodating new devices when they become available.

Vibes of angst over uncertainty radiate from some of the foregoing papers. The system (such as it is a system) for developing devices seems encumbered, maybe even harrassed, and lacks predictability. Given the buffeting to which devices are subjected in regulation, the markets, and the courts, those who invent, develop, and sell these technologies understandably feel uneasy. Gratifyingly little whining comes through in this volume, but occasionally some does emanate from the industry. Chronic whining has been very debilitating to the pharmaceutical industry, and I hope it will be avoided by those who make devices.

Kristine Johnson, speaking from her (unwhining) industry perspective during the symposium, raised concern about five issues: uncertainty in the regulatory criteria; unpredictability of the market; confusion around the bounding provisions for reimbursement; overstandardization of design, to satisfy imposed rules rather than to make devices that would be the most beneficial; and overexpectations of technology assessment for newly devised technologies. All of these issues deserve attention.

INSTITUTIONAL AND INFRASTRUCTURAL ISSUES

No outstanding structural shortcomings are raised in this volume. Several authors wish for a National Science Foundation or other federally supported center of excellence in biomedical engineering or biomedical materials science. At the symposium John T. Watson of the National Heart, Lung, and Blood Institute proposed forming a committee to advise a consortium of federal agencies in identifying opportunities and reducing barriers to innovation. It is hard to evaluate either proposal; their merits might be discussed in future forums.

Apart from a little of the customary grumping about the Food and Drug Administration (FDA), the authors do not generate focused criticisms of regulation. Perhaps the most vexing problem raised is the qualitatively different testing and evaluation problems that medical devices present for regulation, compared with pharmaceuticals. Devices may, for example, be moved into at least a limited experimental clinical market when fewer than a hundred of them even exist. One does not have to be a statistician to recognize the limits this puts on statistical power in evaluating efficacy and safety. Moreover, some device risks reside in potential material failures or design flaws of a sort that only become evident during clinical use; these are extremely difficult to anticipate. Accordingly, design and performance criteria for each kind, or even each model, of device may need to be negotiated between the vendor and the FDA.

When the symposium turned for reassurance to John Villforth from the FDA, he said, in effect, "Don't count on us for too much. A full-dress review of a single device can cost many thousands of dollars and a lot of expertise, and the FDA does not always have the capacity." He said he thought the FDA mainly should serve to pick up sentinel signs and provide feedback to the industry.

Commendably, Frank Samuel argues that what the industry and all of us need is a "competent, efficient, swift, and credible FDA." Surely he is right, and we should hope that the Institute of Medicine (IOM) and other professional organizations will help nourish just those attributes in the agency.

REGULATORY CONTROL VERSUS TORT LIABILITY

Susan Bartlett Foote reminds us that mere compliance with FDA regulations does not insulate a vendor from liability suits. She points out that very different values and criteria underlie the systems of regulation and tort (which are among the feedback loops midway down my scheme of innovation; Figure 1). Regulation is notoriously cumbersome, slow, and costly. Tort cases tend to be capricious, unaccommodating to scientific evidence, and high in transaction costs; moreover, they fail to decouple compensation of those who are harmed from deterrence or punishment of those who cause the harms. Susan Foote's paper outlines a reform scheme that proposes to correct some of these deficiencies in the hybrid regulation-tort system.

Harvey Fineberg offers the chastening observation that, until we accumulate a more robust background record of facts about efficacy and safety of medical devices, tort liability is likely to remain capricious and resist reform.

ECONOMICS

What is the relationship of technologies to health care costs? Understandably, this issue was brought up from the beginning of the symposium to the end. Many individual medical devices carry high price tags, and devices in aggregate add up to a substantial societal burden.

Those costs are far from easy to appraise. What is clear is that simple appraisals can be fallacious. In some ways technologies increase costs; in some ways they decrease costs. Viewed in the micro, they are always expenses. The only way to evaluate them in the larger scheme of things without blowing a mental (or policy) fuse is to view them—like all health care expenses—as investments that return benefits to individuals and society.

The question then transmutes into: What are the costs of these investments, to whom, and what are the paybacks, to whom?

Stuart Altman gives us a solid economics lesson, based on two precepts: (a) There is no free lunch; and (b) economics matter. Further, he asserts two propositions that might be susceptible to empirical examination. First, market elasticity is not simple, and the Econ-1 version of supply-and-demand may well not hold; that is, raising medical costs may not necessarily result in people buying less. Second, because in general in recent years hospitals have experienced rising income from public funds, the income stream has swamped the substitution stream; overall demand simply has increased.

Several authors deal with the economic dynamics—diagnosis-related group (DRG) prospective payment and all that—that shape the market both for standard devices and new ones. No need to go through those arguments here. They are complicated, situation-specific, and periodically need to be examined with respect to given device applications.

Of course, the distributive economic-ethical problem is that whereas medical costs mostly are borne by society's various collective health care financing pools, health benefits from those expenditures accrue to individuals and, in a more diffuse sense, to their families, associates, and society in general.

DIFFUSION

The spread of medical devices throughout the market depends on perceived need, economic considerations, ethical constraints, and a host of other factors covered in the various papers in this volume.

A few problems might be pointed out here. Several authors, starting with Sam Thier, lament the inadequate preparation of physicians and other care providers to evaluate and properly use medical devices, especially new ones. This problem is exacerbated by the rapid rate not only of introduction of new devices but modification of existing ones. Peter Carpenter and Frank Samuel urge devotion of much more attention to development of "software"—such as educational material and training seminars—for users. Doubtless this need will increase as care shifts from hospital into outpatient center and the home (which, incidentally, as Susan Foote has remarked, also is likely to bring new rounds of lawsuits, legitimate and otherwise).

Proper maintenance of devices in the clinic, nursing home, and home is another problem. So is prevention of misuse, misapplication, and outright abuse. Much of the responsibility for these matters will reside with vendors.

Both postmarket surveillance and technology assessment are keys to stable diffusion. The first gathers the essential facts, the second conducts a structured evaluation of the evolving health care prospects. The IOM is involved in several major ways with assessment of medical technology.

Contributions, not mentioned in this symposium, that I think the National Academy of Engineering (NAE) and IOM could make through joint effort have to do with applying decision analysis and related evaluations that grow out of operations research. Engineers already have assisted in this area, such as in optimizing regional blood collection and distribution systems. Although a small and growing band of thinkers is working on these matters, there may well be need for projects here to critique the techniques, develop case analyses, or apply the methods to such problems as systems for collecting data on postmarket failure rates or side effects.

Little can be added here about technology assessment. The endeavor is outlined in the IOM survey, *Assessing Medical Technologies* (Washington, D.C.: National Academy Press, 1985). Although this effort was not discussed in the symposium, everyone seemed to endorse it. A central issue is, how is technology assessment to be paid for? Surely we should channel some sidestream monies from the various reimbursement systems into clinical trials and assessments. How to accomplish this pragmatically is not clear, but it urgently deserves to be discussed. Again, analyzing policies for funding technology assessment may hold a role for IOM, as may nominating devices for high-priority assessment.

How to translate assessment into prescription? More effective ways need to be worked out for applying the feedback from technology assessment to medical strategy and tactics, to actual conditions of device use, to reimbursement schemes, and to the flow of innovation.

CURRENT RESEARCH DIRECTIONS

Leo J. Thomas reviews the exciting variety of bioengineering research possibilities explored in the 1987 National Research Council report, *Directions in Engineering Research* (Washington, D.C.: National Academy Press). These include systems physiology and modeling, neural prostheses, biomechanics, biomaterials, biosensors, metabolic imaging, minimally invasive procedures, and artificial organs.

At the symposium, John Watson urged more research on generic technical questions, to strengthen the whole endeavor. Also he said we need much more work on product reliability. Robert Mann, speaking in part from his experience with natural and artificial hips, emphasized the need to study the fundamental interplay between biochemical factors and biomechanical ones in the body (such as interfacing surfaces, rapidly pressurizing and depressurizing tissues, electromechanical systems, and the like).

Some of this basic and general research is actively being pursued, but some, according to our authors, is not getting the support it needs. No doubt there are openings for further IOM/NAE surveys of research needs, perhaps in quite specialized areas.

Also deserving of Academy attention might be aspects of medical device reliability criteria, reliability testing regimens, and quality assurance. We repeatedly hear assertions that, despite so much general attention to these themes in recent years, with some devices special problems arise that deserve scrutiny and systematization, both to facilitate regulatory evaluation and to ensure quality for ultimate use.

IDENTIFYING NEEDS AND OPPORTUNITIES

In some ways it appears that the most neglected step in the innovation scheme is that last long feedback loop: The one from the ultimate user community back to the start of the whole process.

How, for instance, do practicing physicians, or nursing home operators, or, for that matter, hockey trainers or just folks, who perceive a health problem send the request back to the device enterprise: Please develop such-and-such a gizmo to relieve our problem?

Of course, such feedback may be sensed by that abstract entity we call "the market," or it may be conveyed by various health care providers or advocates, or it may be anticipated in behalf of users by those in a position to innovate.

Here again, there may be roles for the Institute of Medicine and the National Academy of Engineering. From time to time panels might take stock and brainstorm either over health needs in search of technological solution, or over emerging technologies in search of application.

One suspects that initiatives might be defined that would aid our shift toward more effective ambulatory care, home care, and self-care, for example. The congressional Office of Technology Assessment has, by the way, conducted some excellent reviews, such as the recent survey, *Life-Sustaining Technologies and the Elderly* (Washington, D.C.: Office of Technology Assessmnent, U.S. Congress, July 1987).

Sam Thier has remarked that we have not given enough attention to screening techniques and kits, or to rehabilitative devices. Massive-scale screening is getting more attention now, in defending against AIDS and other infectious threats, and in providing employment-related screening. Could IOM/NAE critiquing help?

ENVOI

The only way to make sense of the enormous range of existing devices, variations on those devices, emerging devices, and contemplated future devices is to collect appropriate data and make comparisons.

Once descriptive comparisons are established, the key to broad evaluation is to construe the applications of devices, or indeed, any medical measures, as personal and societal investments.

Always, the ultimate question is, Medical devices *for what?* At the outset of the symposium, no doubt anticipating the frustrations we would experience as we wrestled with this amorphous issue, Sam Thier affirmed straightforwardly: ''The end, of course, is prevention of disease, correction of disease, and rehabilitation from disease.''

Contributors

STUART H. ALTMAN is dean of the Florence Heller Graduate School for Social Policy, Brandeis University, and Sol C. Chaikin Professor of National Health Policy. Dr. Altman is an economist whose research interests are primarily in the area of federal health policy. He serves as chairman of the Prospective Payment Assessment Commission responsible for overseeing the Medicare Diagnostic Related Groups (DRG) Hospital Payment System, chairman on the board of the Health Policy Center at Brandeis University, and as a member of the board of trustees of Beth Israel Hospital. Dr. Altman is a member of the National Academy of Sciences and the Institute of Medicine, where he has served on the governing council. Between 1971 and 1976, Dr. Altman served as deputy assistant secretary for planning and evaluation/health at the Department of Health, Education, and Welfare. From 1973 to 1974 he also served as deputy director for health on the President's Cost-of-Living Council. Dr. Altman holds M.A. and Ph.D. degrees in economics from the University of California, Los Angeles.

PETER F. CARPENTER is executive vice president of ALZA Corporation in Palo Alto, California. Before joining ALZA in 1976, Mr. Carpenter was executive director of Stanford University Medical Center, assistant vice president for medical affairs at Stanford University, and deputy executive director of the U.S. Price Commission. He also served as assistant director of the Center for Materials Research at Stanford University and as program manager for the Advanced Research Projects Agency of the Office of the Secretary of Defense. Mr. Carpenter is currently chairman of the board of directors of the American Foundation for A.I.D.S. Research and cochairman of the Policy Advisory Board to the McGill University Collaborative Programme in Pharmacoepidemiology. Mr. Carpenter received a bachelor's degree in chemistry from Harvard University and an M.B.A. from the University of Chicago.

FLORA CHU is director of medical affairs at the Medical Technology and Practice Patterns Institute in Washington, D.C. At the time of the symposium, she was a medical consultant to the Program in Technology and Health Care in the Institute for Health Policy Analysis at Georgetown University Medical Center. Dr. Chu's research interests include collection of data on the utilization and cost of medical technologies and evaluation of national health policy issues. Dr. Chu holds a bachelor's degree from the University of Pennsylvania and an M.D. degree from the University of Maryland.

HARVEY V. FINEBERG is dean of the Harvard School of Public Health and professor of health policy and management at Harvard University. Dr. Fineberg's interests in health policy include clinical decision making, public health programs, health resource allocation, assessment of medical technology, and dissemination of medical innovations. Among his publications are two jointly authored books *Clinical Decision Analysis* and *The Epidemic That Never Was*, an analysis of the controversial federal immunization program against swine flu in 1976. He is a member of the Institute of Medicine. Dr. Fineberg received his A.B., M.D., and Ph.D. degrees from Harvard University.

SUSAN BARTLETT FOOTE is assistant professor at the School of Business Administration and faculty member of the graduate program in health services management at the University of California, Berkeley. Ms. Foote is author of numerous papers and law review articles on drug and medical device regulation. She is a member of the Forum on Drug Development and Regulation of the Institute of Medicine. She recently served on several Food and Drug Administration panels that reviewed manufacturers' premarket approval applications for newly developed neurological, anesthesia, and general hospital devices and was a member of the advisory panel for the Office of Technology Assessment project on "Medical Technology and DRG's: Evaluating Medicare's Prospective Payment System." Ms. Foote holds B.A. and M.A. degrees in history from Case Western Reserve University and a J.D. degree from the Boalt School of Law at the University of California, Berkeley.

WILSON GREATBATCH is chairman of the board of Greatbatch GEN-AID, Ltd. Mr. Greatbatch is the coinventor of the Chardack-Greatbatch implantable cardiac pacemaker. He is author of many scientific articles and book chapters on medical electronics and "Implantable Active Devices," a book commemorating the twenty-fifth anniversary of the implantable cardiac pacemaker. He is a fellow of the Institute of Electrical and Electronics Engineers, the American Association for the Advancement of Science, the American College of Cardiology, and the British Royal Society of Health and is a member of the National Academy of Engineering. Mr. Greatbatch received his B.E.E. degree from Cornell University and an M.S. in electrical engineering from the University of Buffalo. He has received honorary doctorate degrees from four universities and is named inventor or coinventor on more than 150 U.S. and foreign patents.

RALF D. HOTCHKISS is an independent engineer and designer of products for the handicapped. Mr. Hotchkiss developed many of the innovations in wheelchair design and continues to work on wheelchair improvements under the sponsorship of the Office for Economic Opportunity, the Veterans Administration, and private sources. From 1971 to 1980, he was director of the Center for Concerned Engineering, a consulting group started with the help of Ralph Nader to work on product safety and ethical problems in engineering, where he contributed to public policy efforts related to consumer safety in automobiles and mobile homes and to the development of technologies for the handicapped. He has been a lecturer on wheelchair design and a consultant to wheelchair manufacturers and has given testimony to congressional and conference panels on the subjects of consumer safety, public access for the handicapped, wheelchair safety and dependability. He is author and coauthor of a number of articles and books on consumer safety issues. Mr. Hotchkiss majored in physics at Oberlin College.

ALAN R. KAHN is research professor of electrical and computer engineering at the University of Cincinnati. Dr. Kahn is a physician and private consultant with extensive experience in biomedical engineering applications in the development of new products for clinical use. His research interests include the application of new research in brain physiology, artificial intelligence, human behavior, and communications. From 1982 to 1985, he served on a panel assessing federal policies and the medical device industry for the Office of Technology Assessment of the U.S. Congress. He also helped organize the Alliance of Engineering in Biology and Medicine and served as its third president in 1973. From 1970 to 1977, Dr. Kahn was senior vice president for research and development at Medtronic, Inc., in Minneapolis, Minnesota. Dr. Kahn is a fellow of the Institute of Electrical and Electronics Engineers, the American College of Cardiology, and the American College of Chest Physicians.

WILLIAM W. LOWRANCE is senior fellow and director of the Life Sciences and Public Policy Program at The Rockefeller University. Dr. Lowrance serves on a number of national committees, including the executive committee of the Environmental Protection Agency Science Advisory Board. His research interests include national and international science policy, decisions regarding public health risks, and ethical responsibilities of technical experts. He is author of *Modern Science and Human Values* and *Of Acceptable Risk: Science and the Determination of Safety*. From 1973 to 1975, he served as a resident fellow at the National Academy of Sciences; from 1976 to 1977, as a research fellow in the Program in Science and International Affairs at Harvard University; and from 1977 to 1979, as a special assistant to the under secretary of state. From 1979 to 1981, he taught health and environmental policy as a visiting associate professor in the Program in Human Biology at Stanford University. Dr. Lowrance holds a Ph.D. degree in organic and biological chemistry from The Rockefeller University.

ROBERT W. MANN is Whitaker Professor of biomedical engineering at the Massachusetts Institute of Technology. Dr. Mann's research interests include the biomechanics of synovial joints, the etiology of osteoarthritis, and computer-aided simulation of orthopedic surgery. He is a member of the National Academy of Sciences, the National Academy of Engineering, and the Institute of Medicine and a fellow of the American Academy of Arts and Sciences, the Institute of Electrical and Electronics Engineers, the American Society of Mechanical Engineers, and the American Association for the Advancement of Science. Dr. Mann received his S.B., S.M., and Sc.D. degrees in mechanical engineering from the Massachusetts Institute of Technology.

JOHN H. MOXLEY III was senior vice president for corporate planning and alternative services for American Medical International, Inc., at the time of the symposium. Currently he is president of MetaMedical Inc., a diversified health-care company. Dr. Moxley's research interests are in oncology and the organization and delivery of health care. He is a member of the Council on Scientific Affairs of the American

Medical Association, the Institute of Medicine, the National Academy of Sciences, the American Hospital Association, and the American Association of Medical Colleges. He has served as dean at both the University of Maryland and the University of California at San Diego medical schools, assistant secretary of defense for health affairs at the Pentagon, and clinical associate at the National Cancer Institute. Dr. Moxley received his bachelor's degree from William's College and M.D. degree from the Colorado School of Medicine.

SEYMOUR PERRY is deputy director of the Institute for Health Policy Analysis at Georgetown University Medical Center, where he holds dual appointments as professor of medicine and professor of community and family medicine. Dr. Perry was active in cancer research for 14 years before he was appointed associate director of the National Institutes of Health in 1975 and initiated the formation of the NIH Consensus Development Program, which he headed for the first 3 years of its existence. In 1978, he was appointed an assistant Surgeon General in the Commissioned Corps of the U.S. Public Health Service and designated director of the National Center for Health Care Technology, an agency created by congressional legislation in 1978 to provide assessment of major medical technologies. When the Center was terminated in 1981, he joined the Georgetown University Medical Center. In 1985, he was one of the founders of the International Society of Technology Assessment in Health Care and was its first president. Dr. Perry is a consultant to several government agencies and serves on a number of the advisory and editorial boards. He is a member of the Institute of Medicine and the National Academy of Sciences.

WALTER L. ROBB is senior vice president for corporate research and development of General Electric and a member of the company's Corporate Executive Council. Dr. Robb started his career with General Electric in 1951 as a chemical engineer at the Knolls Atomic Power Laboratory, became head of the Medical Systems Division in 1973, and assumed his present position in 1986. He holds patents related to permeable membranes and separation processes and is widely published in the professional literature. He was vice chairman of the board of regents of the Milwaukee School of Engineering, served on the board of directors of the Health Industry Manufacturers Association, and is a member of the National Academy of Engineering. Dr. Robb holds a B.S. degree in chemical engineering from Pennsylvania State University and M.S. and Ph.D. degrees in chemical engineering from the University of Illinois.

EDWARD B. ROBERTS is David Sarnoff Professor of the Management of Technology at the Massachusetts Institute of Technology's Sloan School of Management. Dr. Roberts' research interests in R&D organizations include the dynamics of health care management and policy, R&D management, technological innovation, entrepreneurship, and new venture activities. He is author of eight books and more than 100 journal articles. In 1958 he became a founding member of the M.I.T. System Dynamics Group, cofounded the M.I.T. Research Program on the Management of Science and Technology in 1961, and became the director of the new interdisciplinary master's degree program in the management of technology in 1980. In 1963 and 1969, respectively, he cofounded Pugh-Roberts Assoc., Inc., an international technology management consulting firm, and Medical Information Technology, Inc. (MEDITECH), a hospital information systems company. In 1982, he became a founding general partner of Zero Stage Capital, a venture capital fund specializing in high-technology startups in the Boston area. Dr. Roberts holds four degrees, including the Ph.D., in engineering, management, and economics from M.I.T.

PENELOPE C. ROEDER was director of corporate planning for American Medical International, Inc., at the time of the symposium. She is currently an independent consultant working with hospitals and physician groups on their strategic planning. Ms. Roeder received a bachelor's degree from Bennington College and an M.B.A. from New York University.

ANTHONY A. ROMEO is chief industrial economist at Unilever in London, England. Dr. Romeo has been a consultant to various private firms and government agencies, including the United Nations, the congressional Office of Technology Assessment, the Federal Trade Commission, the Center for Health Services Research, the National Science Foundation, and the Small Business Administration. From 1971 to 1985, he was on the faculty of the University of Connecticut, where he became professor of economics, with a joint appointment in the Department of Behaviorial Sciences and Community Health. He is author and coauthor of numerous professional articles and two books on the economics of innovation. Dr. Romeo received a B.A. degree in economics from Johns Hopkins University and a Ph.D. degree in economics from the University of Pennsylvania.

LOUISE B. RUSSELL is research professor at the Institute for Health, Health Care Policy and Aging Research and professor in the Department of Economics at Rutgers University. Dr. Russell's research interests in medical policy are related to medical care and the economic effects of demographic trends. Before joining the university, she was a senior fellow in the Economic Studies Program at the Brookings Institution, where she authored three books, *Is Prevention Better Than Cure?*, *Evaluating Preventive Care, The Baby Boom Generation and the Economy*, and *Technology in Hospitals: Medical Advances and Their Diffusion*. She has also published numerous articles on economics and medical care and a book on the federal health budget, based on her work as a research economist both in government and in the private sector. Dr. Russell is a member of the Institute of Medicine and served on the Institute's Committee for the Study of the Future of Public Health. She is also a member of the U.S. Preventive Services Task Force convened by the Department of Health and Human Services. Dr. Russell received her Ph.D. degree in economics from Harvard University.

ARAN SAFIR lives in Cambridge, Massachusetts, and divides his time between the practice of ophthalmology, invention of medical devices, and consultation with industry. His research interests include the optics of the eye, ophthalmic diagnostic and surgical instruments, computers in medicine, and the visual system as an information processor. In addition to holding professional positions in ophthalmology at several medical schools, Dr. Safir participated in numerous committees of the Department of Health, Education, and Welfare during the 1960s and 1970s. From 1975 to 1980, he was director of the Mount Sinai Institute of Computer Science in New York City. He is a fellow of the Academy of Ophthalmology and the American College of Surgeons. Dr. Safir studied electrical engineering at Cornell University, and holds B.S. and M.D. degrees from New York University.

FRANK E. SAMUEL, JR., is president of the Health Industry Manufacturers Association (HIMA). Before joining HIMA in 1984, Mr. Samuel was a partner with the law firm of Dickstein, Shapiro & Morin and held several executive positions in government, including the Department of Health, Education, and Welfare and the Agency for International Development. Mr. Samuel is author of several articles on the health care industry, including several opinion articles. He received a B.A. degree from Hiram College, was a Fulbright Scholar in law and government at the University of Leiden in the Netherlands, and received an Ll.B. degree from Harvard Law School.

SAMUEL O. THIER is president of the Institute of Medicine. Dr. Thier's past appointments include Sterling Professor and chairman of the

Department of Internal Medicine at Yale University School of medicine, vice chairman and professor of medicine at the University of Pennsylvania Medical School, and chief of the renal unit and assistant professor of medicine at Harvard Medical School. Dr. Thier did research at the National Institutes of Health from 1962 to 1964 and served on the director's Advisory Committee from 1980 to 1984. He is author of numerous articles on renal physiology, inherited diseases of the kidney, and kidney stones and is coauthor of a textbook on pathophysiology. Dr. Thier has served as president of the American College of Physicians and chairman of the American Board of Internal Medicine. He received an undergraduate degree from Cornell University and an M.D. degree from the State University of New York at Syracuse.

LEO J. THOMAS is a senior vice president and general manager of life sciences at Eastman Kodak Company and vice chairman of Sterling Drug Inc. Dr. Thomas serves on the board of directors of the Rochester Telephone Corporation and Norstar Bank. He is a member of numerous professional societies, including the American Institute of Chemical Engineers, the American Association for the Advancement of Science, the American Chemical Society, and the Engineering Research Board. He is a member of the National Academy of Engineering and is currently chairman of the Bioengineering Peer Committee. He is also a member of the Board of Chemical Sciences and Technology of the National Research Council. Dr. Thomas received a B.S. degree in chemical engineering from the University of Minnesota and M.S. and Ph.D. degrees in chemical engineering from the University of Illinois.

EDWIN C. WHITEHEAD is founder and chairman of Whitehead Associates, a venture capital and investment company developing biological and chemical products to control or cure disease. Mr. Whitehead is also founder of the Whitehead Institute for Biomedical Research in Cambridge, Massachusetts, and cofounder of Technicon Corporation, where he was chairman and chief executive officer. He holds nearly 20 patents on devices such as the direct-writing electrocardiograph, the portable respirator, the automatic fraction collector, the automatic tissue processor, and automated blood analyzer.

Index